FIT
OVER
FORTY
FOR
WOMEN

LOSE WEIGHT, RECLAIM YOUR ENERGY AND
GET BACK INTO YOUR FAVOURITE CLOTHES

ROB BIRKHEAD

Rethink

First published in Great Britain in 2021
by Rethink Press (www.rethinkpress.com)

Cover image © Shutterstock | OSTILL is Franck Camhi

Contents

Introduction

I speak to many women who have tried everything to lose weight, but since turning forty, nothing seems to be working. They can't seem to get the number on the scales to drop. Many of these women tell me they are losing hope. They think it is part of the ageing process and they will just have to accept it, despite the huge impact it has on their confidence, energy levels, relationships, career and more. It breaks my heart to hear this. The weight loss industry is letting these women down and that's why I wrote this book.

You may wonder why a man in his thirties made it his mission to help women in their forties and fifties lose weight. It began when I was studying a Master's in engineering at the University of Bath. I had always been a skinny teenager and had low self-esteem as a result.

That lead me to start studying nutrition and exercise in my spare time alongside my studies. I used what I learned to change my own body and I was shocked that this changed how I felt. My self-esteem went from rock bottom to starting to believe in myself. I stopped hiding away, came out of my shell and started living life to the fullest for the first time in years. I wanted to help others feel the same way. I realised my true passion was not engineering, but health and fitness.

Instead of pursuing a career in engineering, I started from scratch. I qualified as a personal trainer and started helping everyone and anyone – male and female, young and old. I quickly realised it was easy to get results with men, regardless of their age. It also wasn't difficult to achieve good results with the younger women I coached. For both groups, I could help them to cut back on food or booze, do a bit more exercise – it didn't matter what type – and the weight would start falling off.

It was a different story for the women in their forties and beyond. Nothing I had learned up to that point – high-intensity interval training (HIIT), other forms of cardio, cutting out carbs or hugely reducing calories – seemed to work. The fitness industry had the men and younger women covered, but they had forgotten women who were older, whose hormones were changing and whose bodies didn't respond so easily.

This took me on a journey of discovery. I dedicated the next five years to learning what made these women different, and what I discovered shocked me. The changes happening under the surface for women over forty were beyond anything I'd heard about. Not only were things like menopause not properly understood and accounted for by the weight loss industry, but other changes that happen to women as they get older, such as the stress hormone response, were being ignored. This meant women were routinely being given diets and exercise plans that didn't work. Many made things worse, not better – and I heard from countless women wasting their time, money and energy on a weekly basis, which I felt was unacceptable.

I developed a simple system called the Fit Over 40 method, which helps women in their forties and fifties lose weight by optimising their hormones and get the scales moving again in a healthy and sustainable way. With the Fit Over 40 method, you can lose 1–2 stone every 12 weeks without giving up your favourite foods, having to go to the gym or eating separately from your family. All of this is achievable with a busy full-time career.

This book sets out the step-by-step programme so you can start getting results fast.

The Fit Over 40 programme covers these key steps:

1. What progress to expect

2. The Diet Makeover

3. Low-impact strength training (LIST)

4. Understanding calories

5. The Stress Shield

6. Lifestyle

7. Goal-getting

You will hear from a wide range of women I've worked with over the past decade who've put this programme and these tools into action and transformed their bodies and lives as a result.

By the time you've finished this book, you'll have that understanding and know more about losing weight for women over forty than most personal trainers and doctors. You'll know how to find the time to eat healthily and exercise, keep yourself motivated no matter what, balance your life in all areas, avoid self-sabotage and lose weight in a fast, healthy and sustainable way.

Don't be intimidated by the idea or process of losing weight over forty. Anyone can do it and there is no hidden magic that you can't learn.

PART ONE
A DIFFERENT APPROACH

Women's bodies and hormones change dramatically with age, and these changes start years before menopause.

This means that the strategies that used to work for losing weight in your 20s and 30s actually prevent you from losing weight over 40. They will make you flabbier, more fatigued and increase joint aches and pains.

In order to succeed, you need an approach that works with your changing body and hormones, rather than against them.

In this section you'll discover the extent and impact of these changes, so you not only understand the complex biological shifts that are happening underneath the surface for any women over 40, but also how to work with them to get the scales moving in the right direction again in record time.

1

The Over Forty Weight Gain Trap

The over forty weight gain trap does not happen overnight. It is a snare that tightens over time, and the more you try to wriggle free of it, the more you get stuck. Clothes that fitted perfectly are now tight. Joints creak and ache, and many forms of exercise only make them worse. Lethargy and exhaustion have become the norm and pick-me-ups like caffeine and sugar are now essential to get through the day.

Worst of all, methods that used to work to shift the weight have no effect, and even after a focused week of eating well and exercising, the number on the scale won't budge. Sometimes it even goes up. It's little wonder that many women give up entirely, assuming that it is all part of the ageing process. Not because they don't want to feel fit, healthy and confident, but because becoming tired, old and frumpy seems inevitable.

Many women I've worked with were on the brink of accepting this fate. Their youthful spirit had faded away. Their zest for life turned into a terror of ageing. Special events became a wardrobe nightmare. Holiday photos made trips abroad something to dread. Where was the fit, confident woman who used to love life?

The answer is simple: *methods that work for those in their twenties and thirties don't work for women over forty*. Yet many women keep trying the same things that used to work for them, hoping for a miracle to melt the fat away. This is born out of a fundamental misunderstanding in the fitness industry that not only should women do the same things as men, but that all women should follow the same approach regardless of age. This has cost us dearly in failing health, failing confidence and half-wasted lives.

I call that misunderstanding the over forty weight gain trap. It is rooted in the belief that fitness approaches work the same for all women, which is not the case. Age is a game-changer.

Sowing the seeds

To understand the over forty weight gain trap, let's take a closer look at what happens to women as they get older. If you're like most of the women I work with, the roots of the problem lie years, if not decades, earlier.

In their twenties, they were excited to start their careers. They put everything into it, achieving promotions and climbing the ladder. By thirty, they were on their way to a senior position. That's when things started to change. The responsibility started to mount. Meetings became longer, more frequent and more demanding and the hours and stress mounted up. Their weight occasionally drifted upwards, but it wasn't a huge concern. After a few weeks of eating well and exercising regularly, the weight shifted. But then a spanner was thrown into the works.

For those women who had children, life became complicated with events, classes and clubs to attend, while those without kids often had other caring responsibilities, all while keeping the household in order. On top of that, they continued or returned to full-time work and the number of balls being juggled tripled. The figure on the scales climbed steadily but it now required twice as many gym sessions, and a dramatic change in diet, to rein it in.

Then along came forty. Now family and work are all-consuming. Back-to-back meetings mean lunch is eaten at the computer. After dinner, it's back on the laptop with a glass of wine to finish everything that couldn't be completed in the day. On top of that, ageing parents take more looking after. The feelings of guilt and worry build as they try to please everyone. Inevitably, balls get dropped.

Regular exercise becomes almost impossible because there is no time or energy left. Family and social commitments derail best intentions to eat well and, at the end of a hard week, it's all too easy to say 'yes' to another takeaway. Travelling for work means food choices are limited, schedules are jam-packed and that, combined with jet lag, makes exercise feel impossible. It's exhausting just reading it, let alone living it, yet most of the women I work with are in a similar situation. Exhausted, overworked and over-whelmed. They step on the scale and it reads 1–2 stone higher than it used to. But it's not for a lack of trying.

These women take the same attitude to their fitness as they do their careers. They are high-achievers and, despite being busy, everything in their life is great – with one exception. Nothing they try works anymore to get the scales moving. HIIT, gym classes, running, cycling or swimming. Hiring a personal trainer, join-ing a slimming club, drinking shakes or starting a diet. Cutting out sugar, carbs, fat or alcohol. They put in the work for a month or more but the scales won't budge. Their old clothes don't fit, the belly isn't shrinking, their doctor is still telling them their BMI is too high, yet no one is offering a solution that works.

It's demoralising. They blame themselves. They think the problem is them. That it's their thyroid, their polycystic ovary syndrome (PCOS), their genetics, or maybe they're just lazy. They are on the brink of giving up and accepting that it's all part of getting older. But it's not their fault. The fitness industry is letting women over forty down.

The fatal assumption

In turning forty, you fall victim to the disastrous assumption the fitness industry has been making for as long as it has existed: *that women over forty are the same as women in their twenties and thirties.* This is fatal because it isn't true. It is the root cause of most over forty weight gain in women. Since turning forty, weight goes on more easily and is harder to lose. Most women know this is true.

The fitness industry fails to address this because it assumes all women are the same. The shake diet prescribes the same shake formula regardless of age. The slimming club recommends the same points system and weekly meetings. The trainer takes them through the same workouts and nutrition guidance. The online programme still gives them HIIT, burpees and 1,200 calories a day. The low carb gurus suggest cutting out carbs. These approaches believe that because it works for women in their twenties and thirties, it will work the same for women over forty, which is not true.

This sets women over forty up for failure from day one. The real tragedy is that when someone falls prey to a diet making the fatal assumption, the diet that was supposed to end their battle with weight causes the number on the scales to climb higher than ever before. Suddenly these diets have made food something that can no longer be enjoyed without feeling guilty and afraid afterwards. The exercise that was supposed to eliminate health concerns has left injuries and aches and pains in its wake. Suddenly, the fitness dream turns into a weight gain nightmare.

The career woman stuck in the over forty weight gain trap takes the old fitness approaches that used to work and tries them again. The exercise that used to deliver quick results now does almost nothing for the waistline or the number on the scales. The diets that used to get a stone or more off in a couple of months now barely shift a pound. What's more, they both require a lot of time. Time that the busy forty-plus career woman doesn't have.

The career woman, the mum and the athlete

For many women over forty trying to get fit, there are three people in one: the career woman, the mum and the athlete, all of whom want to succeed. But they are all fighting for the same limited time and energy each day. That's why the problem is so complicated. It's a three-way tug of war that everyone wants to win.

A typical day for many of my clients starts at 6.30am. They get ready as quickly as possible, get the kids ready and get them to school. Now the career woman kicks in. She knows the emails are piling in, there's a day of meetings ahead and no time to waste. 'What about breakfast?' the athlete chimes in. 'How about an omelette and a smoothie and then a quick workout?' But the career woman is already grabbing a coffee. No time for that, she thinks. Food can wait until later. By 1pm, she is starving. She takes a 15-minute lunch break and grabs a wrap and crisps instead. The 2pm slump hits. A coffee and a biscuit should do the trick. 'We'll exercise tomorrow,' says the career woman.

The mum takes over. She rushes home to collect the kids and cook dinner. 'Let's make it something healthy,' the athlete says, even though she hardly knows what a healthy dinner is since she turned forty. 'Pasta and sauce it is, then,' says the mum. Dinner cleared away and chores done, the athlete chimes in again: 'Maybe we can snatch a 30-minute workout now?'

But there is work to do. The mum has a glass of wine in her hand to de-stress while the career woman opens her laptop to finish the day's work on the sofa. An hour or two later, she traipses off to bed, exhausted. But she can't sleep. She feels guilty about work, not spending time with the kids, not exercising and being grumpy with her partner.

If you are familiar with this conflict between the career woman, the mum and the athlete, you will know that you can't be all three; one of them has to lose. It's a three-way battle that no one can win.

The career woman

The career woman has too much to do and too little time to do it. The result? Stress, and lots of it. From the moment she wakes up to the moment she goes to sleep, her mind is on work. When she finally gets a holiday, what happens? A jam-packed week prior to going away, trying to finish everything off. She spends the holiday dreading coming back to a stuffed inbox. She used to take pride in her work but now it's about keeping up on a hamster wheel that spins faster and faster.

This eventually takes its toll:

- Low energy levels make caffeine and sugar essential to get through the day.

- Lack of time means takeaways and ready meals are regular occurrences.

- High stress levels result in turning to alcohol and comfort foods to relax.

- A never-ending to do list means sitting at a desk for 8+ hours a day and no energy to exercise in the evenings.

- Elevated stress hormone levels make losing fat harder.

The same stress that makes it hard to eat well and avoid treats and drinks after a hard day's work also makes it harder to see any weight loss, even if you do avoid them.

But there is hope. The career woman simply needs an approach that keeps stress levels down while still fitting around a busy family life.

The mum

When the career woman returns home, she becomes the mum. The kids need to be fed, the house tidied and bills paid. She dreams of the day the list is done, but it never comes. What happens if her parents or children are unwell? Or the boiler fails? It's enough to send her over the edge. That's when she says 'sod it', orders a takeaway, pours a large glass of wine and proclaims the diet will start again on Monday.

The mum cares for everyone else but forgets herself. There is constant guilt, stress and responsibilities and no time for anything else. There's no time to travel to the weekly slimming club meeting just to step on a set of scales and get a round of applause for losing a pound, never mind scouring the supermarkets for special diet ingredients so she can painstakingly prepare every meal from scratch – meals the rest of the family won't even eat.

Yet this is what many weight loss 'solutions' still prescribe to busy women over forty. The mum needs something that works around the family and can be done quickly and easily. Something that fits around her life, rather than taking it over.

The athlete

Everyone has an athlete inside them. I see this even in clients who have never enjoyed exercise before. The problem is that the athlete inside many of us is confused. This confusion stems from the dieting industry, which suggests that there is a 'best way' to exercise for everyone and that cardio is the best way to burn fat. Whether it's HIIT, running, swimming or cycling, most people think they need to do one or more of these to lose weight, often because a slim friend or social media influencer has told them to.

But here's the thing: staying skinny is easy. You can do almost any kind of exercise and stay skinny. *Losing weight* is a different ballgame. The confused athlete tries jogging because someone told them it is the fastest way to lose weight, despite the fact it makes their knees ache. Then they try HIIT because it's the new 'in' thing, but the knees grumble at the impact, bur-pees leave parts of the body aching that they didn't know existed and star jumps challenge the pelvic floor. This is not sustainable and, when they stop, the results stop (if they ever started).

The same applies to nutrition. Carbs are the enemy, aren't they? Or is it fat? Maybe they should give up sugar or alcohol, or fast for 16 hours a day. The con-fused athlete flip-flops between approaches, hoping that something will stick, but constantly worries they are going to fail. However, it doesn't have to be that way.

An everyday athlete takes care of their body to support the rest of their life. They exercise to get the energy they need to succeed in their career and thrive at home, not to beat their body into submission. They eat in a way that's quick and simple and works around a busy life, and they do it without banning their favourite foods. They understand what drives fitness results and focus on that. They do the minimum work to get the maxi-mum results in a way that's sustainable. If you're an everyday athlete, rather than a 'dieter', you will com-mit to this as a new lifestyle – not just for a few weeks or a few months, but for the rest of your life.

The problem is that the athlete is not only in a battle with themselves. They are in conflict with the mum and the career woman too. Almost all of our clients have a career woman, a mum and an athlete inside them who, if they were equally balanced, would make an incredibly competent individual. Few career women have this balance. The typical over forty woman is divided between the career woman and the mum, with almost nothing left for the athlete. The athlete wakes up with a goal. The mum groans, 'Not again.'

This is a disaster for the body because the balance is out of whack. On a typical day, one of your personalities will be the strongest of the three and control the others. They play their games, fight for their space and sabotage each other continuously. Without all three personalities being given the opportunity, the freedom and the nourishment they need to grow, your body cannot help but mirror your own lopsidedness. It's a war that no one can win until you get the balance right.

CASE STUDY: KERRY

Kerry joined my programme in January 2020. She has two children, is in her mid-forties and works in a high-pressure job in London. Her weight had piled on since having children and she found it impossible between work and family responsibilities to make any time for self-care. What's more, she had a bad back worsened by her weight. She was often in pain and this made her nervous to exercise in case she re-injured it.

Kerry had tried Weight Watchers, swimming, paleo and the Atkins diet, but since turning forty her weight kept climbing. Her son is autistic, which meant these extra challenges would result in giving up whatever diet she was following. Kerry reached a UK size 20 and 100 kg (just under 16 stone). Her health started to impact her career. She struggled to find workwear that fitted, and her boss had given clear signals she was not performing in her job. Kerry knew something had to change.

Within a year of joining my programme, Kerry had lost 30 kg (nearly 5 stone). She feels stronger and more confident and loves her toned arms. She now feels she's setting a great example to her children. She had worried she'd be unable to make time for fitness and self-care, but, with the right approach, Kerry was able to shift the excess weight and get her confidence back without missing out on quality time with her family. She did this because she followed an approach that was right for her – a woman in her forties with a stressful job and family life – an approach that kept stress levels low and fitted around family life rather than taking it over.

I'm excited to share with you the Fit Over 40 method that Kerry and countless other women have used. However, before we go into the process, you need to understand hormones and how they are different for women over forty (and not in the way you might think).

Reflection

To kickstart your journey to becoming fit over forty, it's important to start by setting a goal. Get clear on your starting point and the end goal you're aiming for. Ask yourself the following questions to get clear on what you want to achieve:

- What is your current weight and dress size?

- What approaches have you tried to lose the weight since turning forty? What results have you seen? How long have those results lasted?

- In a year's time, what would success look like for you?

Get a pen and paper and write what comes to mind without judgement. Don't talk yourself out of setting a big goal even if you don't know how to make that goal happen yet – we'll get onto that. For now, just get something down on paper and move on to the next chapter.

Summary

The over forty weight gain trap occurs because women's lifestyles and bodies change significantly after forty, yet the fitness industry doesn't recognise this. Many women attempt to use the same approaches they used in their twenties and thirties to lose weight, but a new approach is needed that takes into account the stresses and strains of family life and a high-pressure job, as well as the biological changes happening beneath the surface.

2

The Hormone Problem:
Stress And Cortisol

The war between the career woman, the mum and the athlete worsens as life gets more complicated and responsibilities mount up. But there are also significant biological changes happening. One key change is menopause. Even though it is more openly talked about nowadays, there is still much misunderstanding about menopause. For example, it is generally thought to happen to women in their fifties, but many changes start years or decades earlier and have a profound effect on the way a woman's body responds to exercise and dieting.

The other change is in how the body deals with stress, which means losing weight as a woman over forty is a different ballgame. Not only are stress levels higher as you get older, but the impact of this stress can trigger a biological switch that makes losing weight almost impossible.

It's the start of a new year and the endless Christmas parties are over. The athlete has been given a chance to combat that winter blubber that's accumulated around your middle. Hope runs high. The athlete is in charge. This year's going to be different. This year you come first. Your diet's had a makeover. There's a ban on booze for January. Crisps, chocolate and biscuits have been replaced by fruit, low fat snacks and rice cakes. Each week, the shopping trolley is now piled high with healthy lean meat, whole grains, fish, fruit and vegetables. Almost every day is a workout day. Either down the gym or jogging through the streets to your favourite tracks.

After a week, you assess your progress. You've stuck to your goals. You've put in the work and feel proud. When you step on the scales, your heart races. The moment of truth. The display flashes and you stare at it, waiting for it to settle. Your heart sinks. One pound down. After all that hard work? You ramp up your efforts, exercising every day during the next week, cutting out snacks and even skipping breakfast. Another week rushes by and you step on the scales again. The number is exactly the same as it was last week. You feel sick to your stomach. It doesn't make sense! Is it the carbs? Too much fat? Maybe I need to do more HIIT? Maybe it's because I'm hormonal? Or is this just part of ageing? In a flash, you realise this year is the same as every year since you turned forty. Nothing seems to work like it should and quickly your motivation fades and you give up.

I'm here to tell you it doesn't have to be like that. When you discover the approaches you've been taking no longer work for your changing body, a new window of opportunity opens. That starts with understanding stress and how it affects the body of a woman over forty.

Stress and cortisol

Many people don't appreciate the impact stress has on the body at a cellular level and how this changes with age. When we get stressed, it triggers our body to release cortisol. Cortisol is the main stress hormone. In short bursts, cortisol has many positive effects. If we exercise, this causes a spike of stress. This short-term stress causes a burst of cortisol to be released, which encourages fat to be released from fat cells. This cortisol release helps your muscles to break down and rebuild stronger than before. These are all good things.

But when cortisol is released all day, the effects are not positive. It becomes 'chronically elevated' in medical terms, and this has negative effects that make losing weight more difficult.

Firstly, it causes insulin resistance. Insulin is a storage hormone, and just like a squirrel that stores away lots of fatty calorific nuts in the autumn ready for winter, insulin resistance means that the body is more likely to store the food you eat as body fat, especially around the middle. Given that we can spend all day working at a desk, barely moving, and our cupboards are usually full of food year-round, this additional fat storage is not necessary or desirable.

Secondly, chronically elevated cortisol levels cause leptin resistance. Leptin is a hormone that controls hunger levels, and when this isn't functioning properly it makes us feel hungrier and crave calorific comfort foods, even after we've already eaten our fill.

Thirdly, chronically high cortisol levels also affect the thyroid, causing it to slow our metabolism. So not only do chronically high stress levels make us want to eat more, they also reduce the amount someone can eat without gaining weight.

These initial effects make stress a significant health challenge in the twenty-first century. If cortisol isn't kept in check, it can turn the body into a fat storing monster that's hard to defeat. But that's just the start.

The impact of ageing

The real challenge comes with ageing. As people get older, their body's reaction to stress, or the stress response, gets more dramatic. This increase in sensitivity to stress isn't the same for both genders. In fact, the stress response in women is three times higher as they age than in men. The knock-on effects of constant stress and high cortisol levels explain why losing weight starts to become harder for busy women as they hit their forties and fifties. Not only are stress levels higher than ever, but the way the body responds to stress becomes more pronounced.

Many modern methods of dealing with stress actually increase cortisol levels. A lot of people like to have a few drinks at the weekend to relax after a hard week, but they don't realise how this affects their cortisol levels. While alcohol numbs the mind, it increases the body's internal stress levels, causing more cortisol to be released.

Lack of sleep also has a huge impact on cortisol levels. Research has found that 97% of adults need 8 hours of sleep a night for their body to function properly – to be energetic, to think clearly and to make good decisions.[1] Yet many cut sleep short, thinking it's a shortcut to getting more done. Then, because they are so tired, they turn to caffeine as a pick-me-up. While drinking coffee may help you stay focused at work, it ramps up your cortisol levels even further.

These lifestyle choices create a hormonal nightmare for many women over forty. Every source of stress – environmental, emotional, psychological, physiological or stress caused by dieting itself – affects our body in the same way, regardless of the source. They all ramp up cortisol levels and make losing weight harder and gaining weight easier.

The sum of all the different stresses on the body is called total stress. If this is too high, cortisol will be elevated to the point where weight loss can become almost impossible. It can lead people to try extreme approaches to lose weight, which may seem like the only way to see results but have the opposite effect for many people. Whether it's cutting calories down to 1,200 a day or fewer, cutting out an entire food group like carbs or fats, or surviving on shakes, everyone wants to find the secret to losing excess weight as quickly and easily as possible. Most people don't understand that eating an extreme diet puts the body under more stress and increases cortisol levels further.

For a young person, this may work. Life is less stressful and less complicated and the body is better able to deal with elevated cortisol levels. For women in their forties and beyond, these extreme diets can stress out the body so much that the weight won't shift and it will send hunger and cravings through the roof.

I see this all the time with modern exercise trends – HIIT, spinning, intense gym classes, brutal personal training sessions or long runs. The thought is that the harder you work and the more you sweat, the more fat you burn. This may be true for those in their twenties and thirties, but when the stress response is heightened in women over forty, this can be a disaster. Combine an extreme diet with high-intensity exercise and a stressful life, and the total stress on the body gets too high for too long and losing weight becomes almost impossible.

It's a vicious cycle. You try harder to lose weight and see fewer results the harder you try.

Perimenopause and menopause

Changes to the female sex hormones occur well before officially hitting menopause.

Clinical menopause – the medical definition – is when a woman hasn't had a period for 12 months straight. The word menopause actually means your last menstrual period – 'meno' refers to your menstrual cycle and 'pause' literally means stop. When menopause occurs, the ovaries stop producing eggs and, as a result, the levels of the sex hormones oestrogen and progesterone drop significantly. This is still widely thought to only happen to women in their fifties, but it can happen many years earlier. More importantly, this doesn't happen suddenly, but gradually over time. As renowned menopause expert, Dr Louise Newson, says:

'During a natural menopause, our ovaries
won't suddenly stop working, rather they slow

down over time. I have treated women who have experienced symptoms for a couple of months, others have been plagued for several years or even decades before their periods finally stop.'[2]

This time before menopause, when changes are occurring but periods haven't completely stopped, is called perimenopause. The word perimenopause means near menopause. How near differs from woman to woman, but it can happen 10 years before menopause in some cases, which means it's not uncommon for women in their late thirties and forties.

The side effects of these hormonal changes are more significant than many women are aware of. Many assume the effects they are experiencing are just part of the stresses and strains of life. Others may have symptoms so mild they don't realise they are caused by hormonal changes. But both have one thing in common – they notice that losing weight is more challenging than it ever was before.

So, there are significant changes happening internally for women over 40, and to be able to lose weight successfully, fitness approaches need to evolve to work with these changes, rather than against them. Unfortunately, most diets and exercise programmes don't follow this principle. Instead, most operate according to what works for most people as opposed to what works for the specific person they are working with. Diet plans want the most dramatic results from the people who can see the quickest changes (typically those in their twenties and thirties), so that they can share the results and enrol more paying customers onto the diet as quickly as possible.

This dooms the over forty woman before she has even started. This is due partly to the effects of cortisol but can be further exacerbated by the changes in female sex hormones happening during perimenopause. Understanding each hormone, and how it affects the body's ability to lose weight, is critical to discovering why most women over forty struggle to lose weight and ensuring that you won't.

Oestrogen

Oestrogen is the best-known of the female sex hormones and has the most advantages. It inhibits visceral fat storage and prevents fat being stored around the middle and around your organs. This type of fat has the most health risks, predominantly from heart disease, so oestrogen is said to protect women from heart disease.

It increases levels of leptin, which is the hormone that stops you feeling hungry, so it helps reduce cravings and comfort eating. It increases insulin sensitivity, which makes it easier for your body to process carbs and prevents it storing them as fat, which is the opposite of the effect stress and cortisol have on these hormones. Oestrogen also increases dopamine and serotonin. These are known as the 'happy hormones' and they help you feel energetic, content and positive. Lastly, oestrogen helps prevent inflammation, which protects your joints and keeps them working smoothly and without pain.

In summary, it helps the female body stay healthy and keeps you feeling good in mind and body. However, these benefits are effectively reversed during peri-menopause and menopause (unless you take HRT that replaces the missing oestrogen). As oestrogen levels fall during menopause, the balance between oestrogen and testosterone changes, and testosterone becomes relatively higher. This leads to increased visceral fat storage, which contributes to the middle-aged spread that forms in many women in their forties and beyond.

When oestrogen drops, levels of the hunger hormone leptin drop with it. This means you'll feel hungrier. Combine this with the leptin resistance that comes with high cortisol levels and it's a double whammy, making comfort foods more tempting and less filling. This is made worse due to dopamine and serotonin levels falling. Oestrogen boosts these happy hormones, but when it drops during menopause, mood and energy levels can drop too. This means sugary foods become even more appealing for a quick pick-me-up.

Insulin sensitivity also drops when oestrogen levels drop during menopause. The body becomes more likely to store fat, especially from processed carbs like sugary treats. Again, when combined with high stress levels, the increased cortisol caused by stress also creates insulin resistance, which makes fat storage even more likely, especially from sugary foods.

Careful consideration needs to be given to food choices and lifestyle changes during menopause. The hormonal changes happening beneath the surface make it easier to over-eat and harder to lose weight. Decreased oestrogen makes cravings worse and the body can't deal with certain foods in the way it used to. It's a hormonal headache and unless it's treated in the right way, no matter what you do, the weight will not budge.

The most tragic part of perimenopausal weight gain is that most women are not aware of what they are up against. Many women are strong-willed and determined not to be beaten. They try a new diet with a vengeance, convinced they are not working hard enough and are fully committed to doing whatever is necessary to make it work. They eat separately from the family. They go to three different shops a week to get all the right foods. They order shakes and meal replacements. They give up their favourite foods and alcohol. They sign up to the gym or download another dozen workout apps and commit to doing them every day. They give it everything they have but it doesn't work.

Does this sound familiar? This condition of over forty weight gain dominates the lives of women across the globe. But there is a better way. Inside my Fit Over 40 programme, we use a system called the F3 Formula, which is explored in the next chapter.

CASE STUDY: CATHERINE

Catherine battled with hormonal challenges for almost a decade. She was fifty-two, with two children at university, and she worked as a communications manager. She had gained weight steadily for the past 10 years. On top of a stressful job, the menopause had resulted in her piling on the weight. She had tried HRT, which helped with some menopause side effects, but it didn't get the weight off. Occasionally she'd do gym classes and try to eat healthily. Sometimes she'd lose a few pounds but she always regained it. She had to buy size 14 clothing as nothing she owned fitted properly anymore. She hated her arms and belly, and her thighs would chafe in hot weather. She was shocked to find out she was pre-diabetic, but nothing she did seemed to work.

The good news is that we were able to change all that. Following an approach that avoided over-stressing the body, Catherine quickly lost 10 inches in body fat from her waist, hips and legs, and a stone in weight, and she was able to ditch the size 14 clothes. She now wears a size 10. More importantly, she got the all-clear for diabetes. Using our F3 Formula, Catherine was able to rebalance her hormones and her life in general, which got the number on the scales dropping quickly and easily.

Reflection

This exercise will help you figure out whether your current approach is too stressful.

Step 1: Deduct your age from sixty-five (eg if you're forty-seven, you get eighteen points). This is called your stress reserve (remember, your body's stress response increases with age, and three times more as a woman). Note: If you're over 65, your stress reserve will be zero.

Step 2: Use the following questions to work out your current stress levels.

1. How would you rate your stress levels at work out of ten (zero = a total breeze and ten = pulling your hair out)?

2. How would you rate your stress levels at home out of ten?

3. Have you tried any of the following to lose weight recently?

   - HIIT
   - Gym classes

- Spinning

- Running

- Eating 1,200 kcal or less

- Shake diets

Score yourself five points for each one you've tried recently.

4. How many hours fewer than the recommended 8 hours of quality sleep a night are you getting? Eg if you get 7 hours' sleep, score yourself one.

5. If you are going through menopause, score yourself an additional five points, otherwise score yourself zero points for this question.

Add up your scores from questions 1–5. This will give you an estimate for the total stress on your body.

Total stress levels: ___

Now compare that to your stress reserve that you worked out in Step 1. Is your total stress level higher or lower than your stress reserve?

If your total stress level is higher than your stress reserve, it's likely your cortisol levels will be too high and making it difficult to lose weight. You will need to reduce the total stress on your body, using the methods covered in the next chapter.

Summary

There are two key hormonal changes that happen for women over forty:

1. Increased stress response

2. Menopause

These changes can make losing weight difficult when using the wrong approach. Most quick fix diets and fitness programmes don't take these into account and make things worse, not better.

To escape the over forty weight gain trap, an approach is needed that works with these changes, rather than against them. One that keeps the body's internal stress levels low and doesn't disrupt hormones that make losing weight more difficult for women over forty.

3
The F3 Formula

What has your family life got to do with your weight? The majority of diets and fitness plans are focused on the wrong thing. They deal with the weight problem in a vacuum. They assume that you just need a new way to eat, move a bit more, do a few workouts and burn a few calories and the weight will fall off. That may be great in theory, but they miss out why people *don't* do those things. They take a one-dimensional view of fitness, which leads most people to fail.

A holistic view must be taken because everything in your life is intertwined. It doesn't happen in a vacuum. Remember the last time you had a row in your relationship. You were probably fuming. That night, was the chocolate, the wine or the crisps more tempting?

Or maybe your children were unwell and you had to juggle meetings and phone calls while caring for the kids until they felt better. Then there are those weeks when you haven't had a second to eat lunch and you spend your evenings working. This is a vicious cycle that many women are stuck in for years. Even if they knew what was best for them in terms of diet and exercise, they'd struggle to actually do it.

Simply *knowing* what to do isn't enough. Eating well and exercising regularly won't happen if everything else stops them from happening. The best fitness approach isn't just one that works for you biologically – it's also the one that works with the rest of your life. One that helps manage the stresses of family and work life.

As Ryan Holiday says in his bestselling book, *The Obstacle is the Way*, 'The only guarantee, ever, is that things will go wrong. The only thing we can use to mitigate this is anticipation. Because the only variable we control completely is ourselves.'[3]

The older you get, the more complicated life gets and the more responsibility you take on in and out of work, the more things there are to go wrong. Pressure and stress can be at an all-time high with no way of releasing them.

The weight loss industry's dirty little secret

When I launched my company TRINITY Transformation in 2014, I studied the science of fitness and losing weight in a healthy and sustainable way. Based on this research, I built a programme that was personalised for clients in every way we thought necessary. I expected their results would be unprecedented. But despite giving people the best possible approach, their results remained almost the same. It wasn't that the programme didn't work, it was that clients struggled to put it into practice consistently enough to see any lasting change. Clients hit the 'sod it' button mid-week after a stressful time at work, only to undo all their hard work over the weekend and start from scratch every Monday. This would happen over and over, and they lost more motivation each time, until eventually their hope faded away.

This constant battle is considered normal by many diets. They say that's just how it is. That if someone loses weight and they regain it all shortly afterwards, that still counts as a success. To me, this is unacceptable. My clients put their faith in me to deliver a result. They want a permanent change in their health and fitness, not a temporary blip. If that weight is regained, it is not a success story.

Many people blame themselves – they assume they can't have tried hard enough or didn't have enough willpower. They don't realise that the approach wasn't right for them in the first place. It made their stress levels worse and further disrupted their changing hormones, making it harder to lose weight than before. It also didn't take into account the external influences on their fitness results. Fitness, family and fun are all part of the same puzzle that must be solved as a whole, not individual games to be played separately. Without this level of clarity, the game is being played blind. People try to solve all three areas without finding a way to fit them together.

My team and I went back to the drawing board. After years of trial and error, we realised that to achieve lasting results, a balance needs to be found between three key pillars: fitness, family and fun. This would create a stable platform for our clients to transform every aspect of their lives. They'd find more energy to thrive at work. They'd walk into meetings with their head held high, wearing what made them feel good. They'd come home and feel present with their children and partner and no longer need to turn to booze or comfort eating. Their joints would no longer ache, they'd wake up each day fizzing with energy and they'd have a spring in their step.

The F3 Formula became our top priority. This system has been the secret to the success of our clients, many of whom were on the brink of giving up and accepting the weight gain and lack of results was just part of getting older.

The fitness pillar

When you want to get fit, you need to know the best thing to do and how to do it. What to eat and when to eat it. What type of exercise to do and how much. How much water to drink, what supplements to take and so on. Before we get into the specifics of what kind of programme works best to get and stay fit over forty, we need to understand the overall philosophy behind it, what we're trying to achieve and why. Only then can we dive in and look at the specifics. When it comes to the fitness pillar of the F3 Formula, there are three things we need to consider:

- Stress

- Injury

- Time

You now understand how managing stress levels is key to losing weight for good over forty. This means managing stress from work and family life and also managing the stress on the body from a fitness point of view.

There are two types of people in terms of fitness:

1. **The overdoer:** someone who stresses the body through over-exercise and extreme dieting to the point where weight loss becomes difficult. Cortisol levels are through the roof and body fat

will not be beaten into submission. They try to outdo everyone else in the gym, or they follow fitness programmes to the letter, not knowing they are designed for those in their twenties and thirties. They try to eat 1,200 calories a day or survive on shakes. Whatever the extreme approach is, the result is the same – despite the sweaty workouts and constantly feeling hungry, nothing happens.

2. **The underdoer:** someone who barely moves all day, due to copious amounts of desk work to get through. There is not enough activity to compensate for even a moderate intake of food. Either they have to starve themselves to see any kind of change on the scales, which over-stresses the body as it senses it's starving and cortisol levels become too high, or they do nothing. They eat healthily in moderation but their weight doesn't budge.

I call this dichotomy the Goldilocks principle. In the folk tale, Goldilocks tries the three bears' porridge: one that's too hot, one that's too cold and finally she finds one that's just right. The Goldilocks principle applies to fitness, too. With the overdoers, the approach is 'too hot' and too hard. It's over-stressing the body, sending cortisol levels skywards and locking the number on the scales in place. It also applies to the underdoers. Their approach is 'too cold', too soft. It doesn't create enough stimulus to get the body to change.

What the body needs is a fitness approach that's 'just right'. One that gets the metabolism going, tightens and tones the body but protects the joints and keeps stress levels moderate, so cortisol doesn't block weight loss. It has to provide enough food so the body doesn't sense it's starving and stress levels remain healthy, but not so much that the body stops burning body fat for energy. It's a fine balance and once struck it means weight starts to fall off quickly.

Many women have little spare time to dedicate to their health and fitness, but most fitness approaches are demanding of people's time. They require finding complex ingredients, travelling to slimming clubs just to step on a set of scales, spending hours in the kitchen prepping meals, many of which won't be eaten by the rest of the family, or going to the gym five or six times a week. All this is taking from what little time they have with their family.

In reality, most fitness 'solutions' are inefficient because they are unspecific, which means they take up far more time than is really needed to deliver a good result. They are blunt and ineffective and rely on people struggling to get a result. They may achieve the job eventually, but it will take a *lot* of time and effort.

When a fitness approach is tailored to an individual – taking into account their age, weight, height, body fat percentage, body type, hormonal position, health issues and dieting history – it can achieve stunning results in a short space of time. Clients on my programme usually work out three times a week from home and eat normal foods that the whole family can enjoy. They typically lose 1–2 stone and one to two dress sizes in 12 weeks or less.

However, there's more to the F3 Formula than just the fitness side.

The family pillar

Most weight loss 'solutions' ignore the fact that eating and exercise are influenced by other areas of life. They give you detailed strategies for what to eat and how to exercise, but when it comes to dealing with a family disaster, ill parents or a difficult time in a relationship, you're on your own. As people get older, their responsibilities increase, whether it's due to starting a family or having to care for ageing parents. Many of the women I work with are caring for their partner, their children, their dog, their parents and even their parents-in-law. They need a way to dissipate the stress and slow down. Otherwise they will start every week with good intentions but end the week back where they started.

There are three key sources of family stress:

- Children

- Parents

- Relationships

We can shorten this to CPR. Usually, CPR is a lifesaver, but on the path to becoming fit over forty it can be the death of someone's fitness dreams.

Children

Children can be key in the struggle to lose weight and keep it off. Everything revolves around them. Being a mum is a full-time role with little let up. Whatever stage of life your children are at, if that stress isn't managed, it can derail the best intentions to eat well and exercise.

On top of that, mothers can lose their independence and identity through the process of caring. They forget how to prioritise themselves. They have come last for so long that it requires a lot of effort to get back into the groove with self-care. Many women I speak to want their children to be healthier, exercise more, look after their mental and physical health and have more self-worth. In the process of trying to be the best mother, they forgot to do these things for themselves. They are so absorbed in work and parenting that they don't look after their own health. They are constantly stressed and frantic, yet they expect their children to behave differently. My meditation teacher,

Arjuna Ishaya, suggests that all parents should 'be a lighthouse', meaning to stand tall and lead by example.[4] If we apply this to physical and mental health, this means doing whatever you need to be fit, healthy and happy so that your children will follow in your footsteps.

In the F3 Formula, we use a tool called the Stress Shield, which we will come to later. This releases the stresses of family life. It allows you to stay calm, so you can be consistent with healthy eating and exercise choices but also demonstrate to those around you how to navigate these times without self-destructing or abandoning your own self-care.

Parents

Parents can be another significant source of stress. You might have interfering in-laws or older parents whose health is declining. Visiting parents in hospital or at care homes can present limited choices, with often only a basic canteen loaded with beige foods to choose from. These scenarios often lead people to think that there is no point in continuing if they can't do it perfectly.

Without the tools to deal with these thoughts and challenges, many people go off course. They might make poor food choices or skip their planned exercise. When this happens regularly, it can quickly become a downwards spiral. One bad day can become two, three, then, 'Sod it, I'll start again next Monday.' You'll progress one week and then undo all that hard work the next. Even with the best fitness programme in the world, this will never work. You've got to stay consistent.

It is essential you have the tools needed to manage that stress, so that when things start to slip, you can dig yourself out of the downwards spiral and get back on track as quickly as possible.

Relationships

The last key source of family-related stress is relationships. Minor issues like arguments can be resolved quickly, but they can still lead to poor eating habits or sabotaging a workout. The most challenging are deep-rooted relationship issues that cause growing resentment from years of snide comments, gradually growing apart from your partner, or even the implications of a divorce or an affair. Relationship problems can be all-consuming and can wipe out health and fitness aspirations.

Relationships can be challenging, even at the best of times. In many cases, people try to suppress the problems and push them to one side. But this builds resentment, worry, frustration, fear and even anger over time. This can lead people to increased drinking and emotional eating, which takes its toll on the body and forces it to store these excesses as body fat.

Relationship problems can leave a trail of destruction that reaches much further than the relationship itself.

Challenges in a relationship are normal. To lose weight successfully, it is important to have the tools to tackle any relationship challenges. You also need ways to keep the spark alive in a relationship after marriage and children, otherwise boredom creeps in. We suggest various ideas in the F3 Formula, from weekly 'date nights', to goal-setting, to using the Stress Shield to process problems and deal with them in a more productive way.

The F3 Formula is a holistic solution to a holistic problem that takes into account all the sources of stress and provides you with tools and systems to stop anything from derailing your fitness journey. It allows you to thrive at work and at home but stops those two things from taking over and putting the brakes on your fitness progress.

CASE STUDY: PATRICIA

Patricia's weight was out of control. She had hit her fifties and, combined with the hormonal changes around menopause, she had a lot of stress in her family life and at work. Patricia was the director of her own award-winning landscape gardening business. She put in long hours and worked most weekends. When she wasn't in the office or travelling between clients, she was at home looking after her two daughters. Then, when her younger daughter was fourteen, she was diagnosed with refractory epilepsy, a form of untreatable epilepsy. Patricia's daughter was in and out of hospital for the next few years. This took its toll on Patricia and her husband and their solace lay in a bottle of wine.

Around the same time, her brother died suddenly and then Patricia's mother had a stroke. For the next two years, Patricia juggled looking after her mother, working, being a parent and a partner. Her stress levels were out of control and the only way she coped was with food and drink. The weight piled on. She had a bad back, a frozen shoulder and even spent 3 months in a wheelchair, her body too worn out to carry her own weight.

In 2015, after nine traumatic years, Patricia decided enough was enough. She needed to make herself the priority again. She had never been so heavy. She felt tired and sluggish, had no energy and her self-confidence was rock bottom. She started an American programme that focused solely on diet and she started eating a little better, but she knew she had a lot more to lose. She got in touch with me at TRINITY Transformation as she wanted to accelerate her progress and do something that focused on more than just a quick fix diet.

Patricia followed the approach outlined in this book, including a tailored nutritional and exercise programme that worked with her hormones rather than against them, and the weight started to come off. But the real change was in how Patricia used our mindset tools like the Stress Shield to deal with stresses that had previously been the primary cause of her eating, drinking and subsequent weight gain. With this approach, Patricia went from a size 14 to a size 10, then kept going and reached a size 8.

She had learned a valuable lesson. 'Don't keep restarting it. Don't keep missing weeks because life's always going to throw rubbish at you and you're just going to have to get on with it. The only thing that's going to make you feel better is you and how you deal with the problems that life throws at you.'

Family life will throw you curveballs. To lose weight and keep it off in your forties and fifties, these things must not be left to chance. You must learn the tools to take care of these family challenges, or they will take care of you and your fitness results.

The fun pillar

How can fun be related to your fitness results? Isn't having fun part of the problem? This chapter isn't about robbing you of your social life or having to give up drinking or enjoying a meal out. Fun, in the context of the F3 Formula, comes down to three things which are completely overlooked by most fitness plans and diets but are key to good results, especially long term:

- Me time

- Rest

- Recovery

Me time

Many of my clients say that their only regular source of 'fun' is food and drink. Takeaways, meals out, snacks and wine on the sofa or celebrating birthdays with cakes, treats and perhaps a bottle of champagne. Other than that, their life is only about work – both in their job and around the house. Over the years, the fun evaporates. Those things that were an escape from everyday life are now gone. Those things that made you *you* vanished almost overnight without you noticing it was happening. Hobbies are a distant memory. Work and family life have eaten into the other aspects of fun: rest and recovery.

Rest

Sleep starts to suffer. Working late into the evening means that getting off to sleep is now a daily battle. You browse social media, read the news or message friends later into the night, trying to justify it as quality 'me time'. When you do sleep, it is broken. In becoming that high-achieving career woman and best possible mum, fun, rest and recovery are sacrificed.

In the short-term, this may be necessary to raise children and to earn enough to support the family's needs. In the long run, it will have a profound effect on your physical and mental health. Many clients tell me they no longer recognise themselves, and not just physically. They feel they have lost themselves along the way.

A large part of this is because the fun, rest and recovery in their life have been eliminated. They have been eroded over the years until nothing is left except for food and drink, whether it's to celebrate, commiserate, pick themselves up or unwind and escape. This is because fun, rest and recovery are *fundamental human needs*. If you don't give your body and mind the fun, rest and recovery it needs, it will seek them out in the easiest way possible – through food and drink. These won't fill the void in the long term and they'll leave you feeling unhealthy, lethargic and unfulfilled.

Recovery

For the modern working woman, rest, enjoyment and fun are seen only as a reward for success. Only when you've got to the goal do you deserve to rest, do something just for you and enjoy yourself again. But the goal posts are always moving. Before you've finished your current project, there are another two in your inbox. That reward – that rest you always promise yourself – never comes.

But fun and rest are not rewards for success. They are *prerequisites* for success. To achieve the life you desire, a life that's fulfilling, exciting and bright, you must first get the rest and recovery you need so you can thrive. Start living and looking after yourself now before it's too late. This is the final piece of the puzzle and is the hidden key to your transformation. It's time to stop putting yourself last.

CASE STUDY: LOU

Lou couldn't stop giving in to emotional eating. If she got stressed or was busy working until 11pm, she'd eat. 'Food became comfort,' she said. 'If I was bored, lonely or putting off going to bed because I couldn't sleep, eating was just something to do. We worked really hard on mindset at TRINITY, where you talk about all these things. I learned to say, "OK, so when this thing happens in my life, food can't be the answer. I need to solve it in some other way."' Over time, Lou learned there were times when she had to put herself first. 'As a working mum, it's difficult to stand back and say, "No, actually, I'm going to put myself first this time, because I matter and if I don't, this is the consequence," and the consequence for me was emotional eating.'

Lou started off at a size 22 and a year later was a size 8. Her BMI has come down from 40 to 22 and she has lost over 7.5 stone.

Reflection

Use the F3 Formula to help you figure out what areas of your life need the most improvement. If this shows your life is out of balance, it can help to explain why problems like emotional eating or drinking are occurring and show which areas need improving to eliminate these problems.

To do this, rate each of the following areas out of ten.

Fitness

- Fitness levels
- Body confidence

Family

- Relationship with your partner (or how happy you are on your own, if you're single)
- Relationship with your children (or friends, if you don't have children)

Fun

- Me time
- Daily energy levels

What are your bottom three areas (those with the lowest score)? Focus on improving these areas first, and everything else will improve with it.

Summary

To successfully lose weight over forty, your life needs to be in balance. A holistic approach is required, which doesn't just focus on eating and exercise and making that fit around the rest of your life, but equips you with the tools and tactics to stop work and family life from derailing your fitness journey.

4

The Seven Success Strategies To Get Fit Over Forty

Over the last 10 years, I've identified seven essential ingredients. Getting fit over forty, and staying that way long term, is something that eludes many people because they are missing one of these key strategies. Miss any one, or remove them too soon, and you are doomed to failure.

These ingredients are divided up into two areas:

- The four phases of a lifetime transformation

- The three essential motivators

The four phases of a lifetime transformation

Most basic diets dive in at the deep end. They give you everything upfront and you have to digest it all in one go, which leads to two inevitable outcomes. They over-simplify it to make it manageable, which won't deliver results for those over forty, or they give you everything you need in one huge lump. Work out every day, cut out these foods, eat at these times, eat this much protein and this many carbs, do these stretches in the evening, put yourself first, learn to love your body and so on. It's overwhelming and people often give up within the first 2 weeks.

Neither approach works. What works much better is to break the process of getting fit over forty down into bite-sized chunks.

Stage 1: Reboot

Duration: 12 weeks

Reboot is about breaking bad habits and building new ones. Trying to build new healthy habits while you are stuck in unhealthy patterns won't cut it. Try to do that and you will find yourself constantly undoing your hard work, which kills your motivation when you don't see results. If you always reach for the biscuit jar or a bottle of wine when bored or stressed, you will easily wipe out the positive effects of any new healthier habits. It's like trying to use an old computer that runs slow and constantly crashes. No matter how hard you try to get things done, it will keep going wrong. You must turn it off and reset it so it works properly again and you can get things done productively.

In the Fit Over 40 programme, we start by resetting the most basic habits when it comes to nutrition and exercise. These will deliver the maximum results for the minimum effort.

This must be done across the F3 Formula – fitness, family and fun – not just in the area of fitness, so that the approach fits around your life, works with your changing hormones rather than against them and avoids stress overwhelming and derailing your fitness efforts.

This rebooting process typically takes 6-12 weeks. By then, you will have built up each habit week by week and put these things into action consistently. Then it's time to move onto the next key stage to success: reframe.

Stage 2: Reframe

Duration: 12 weeks

It's all well and good losing a stone or two, but unless you can keep it off long-term, what's the point? Most people can lose a bit of weight, but they can't keep it off. They're forever taking one step forwards and two steps back, and even if they know what to do, they stop doing it when life throws them a curveball.

In order to stop this happening we must make better decisions. When we make better decisions consistently, we get very different results in our life, and weight loss comes much more easily. As discussed later in the Stress Shield part of the programme, all our decisions start with our thoughts, and if we can change our thought process we can change our results.

The reframe part of the process is all about rewiring your brain to eliminate negative thinking and self-sabotage, so you can stop stopping, and start seeing consistent progress no matter what life throws at you. We use a tool called the Thought Transformer to do this which we'll discuss in the Stress Shield chapter of this book.

It takes around 12 weeks to master this process, and in that time you should be able to lose another 1–2 stone.

Stage 3: Reverse

Duration: 12 weeks

Once you've reached your goal weight, you can't just go straight back to eating normally. This is a mistake many people make and they quickly regain the weight they lost, and often more! The reverse process is critical to ensure this doesn't happen and you keep off all the weight you lose.

Your body is smart, and when you reduce the amount of calories you're eating, which is essential to lose weight, it will naturally slow your metabolism down. If you drastically reduce your calorie intake, which we don't recommend doing, especially as a woman over 40, this will happen very quickly. If you reduce your calorie intake slowly and carefully, your metabolism will take much longer to slow down, but it will still slow down to a degree.

To avoid regaining weight you must rebuild your metabolism doing something called reverse dieting. This is where you carefully increase your calorie intake over a period of 6-12 weeks. Do this properly and many people actually lose more weight, and can then eat more normally and keep the weight off with ease.

Stage 4: Maintain

Duration: 12 weeks and beyond

There are two elements to this final stage. The first part is about repeating your new habits long enough for two things to happen.

Firstly, the habit needs to be repeated enough for it to become ingrained so that it no longer requires effort to keep up. Charles Duhigg, bestselling author of *The Power of Habit*, says that the time it takes for a habit to become automatic depends on how complex it is. This can take between 18 and 254 days, with an average of 66 days for it to become automatic.[5] Shifting eating and exercise habits for good will be in the upper end of this range as they are complex habits.

Just like in the gym, the more repetitions you do of a particular movement, the stronger that muscle gets. The same thing applies to your overall weight loss goals. Repeating what works enough times to get the results you want won't give you the dopamine hit that buying another fitness plan can do, but it's where the majority of long-lasting results happen. It's what it takes to make a truly life-changing transformation. Once you've made that transformation and achieved your goals, the focus shifts to maintenance and how to keep the weight off long term.

Maintenance is not as strict as repetition. You don't have to track what you're doing quite so closely and there is much more flexibility. That's because your body wants to stay exactly as it is. This is what makes losing weight hard, but it makes maintenance a lot easier. The trap most people fall into when trying to maintain is that they swing from doing the right things to lose weight to doing exactly what they did before. They stop putting themselves first, stop buying healthy food, stop trying to achieve a balance with alcohol and start drinking regularly again. They stop using mindset tools to manage their stress levels. They get rid of the coach who was keeping them accountable. You might be able to eat out a bit more and have a couple more drinks. But completely stopping exercise, overeating and drinking too much only has one outcome – going back to square one.

That's why this maintenance phase is so important. It's about finding an approach that avoids the rebound most people see after doing quick fix diets. A maintenance strategy looks different for every person and is about what they feel confident doing long term that will maintain their results.

These four phases are key to achieve a lifetime transformation – to lose the excess weight and keep it off for good. They are not the overnight transformation touted by many quick fix diets. To lose weight and keep it off requires repetition. It means consistently using what works for as long as it takes to get the weight off – typically 12 weeks to a year depending on how much weight someone's got to lose. Even then, once you've lost the weight and you are happy with your figure, you must keep up some level of consistency to avoid regaining the weight.

This will take motivation, and we'll get onto that now with the three essential motivators.

The three essential motivators

It can seem noble to attempt to lose weight alone. It might even appear to save you money, but if that approach had worked, you would already be in shape. I learned this the hard way. At university, I had my friend and now business partner, Ben, to work out with. We kept each other accountable to stick to our exercise and healthy eating regime, and it was easy to stay on track. But then I returned to my hometown and it was just me dragging myself out of bed each day to do a workout. If I wanted to give up, I could. I became less fit and more out of shape. I knew what to do but I wasn't doing it consistently. I lost all enthusiasm for my health and fitness. Eventually, I signed up at my local CrossFit gym and I've been a member ever since. They told me what to do so I didn't always have to figure it out myself. Then they held me accountable to follow through with the plan. Most importantly, I was surrounded by likeminded people, which meant when I hit a problem there were others struggling with it and we could work through it together.

So even I – an experienced personal trainer with over a decade of experience – don't write my own fitness programmes or keep myself accountable. I realised that in order to succeed, I too needed three essential motivators: accountability, support and community.

Essential motivator 1: Accountability

Accountability is simple. It's basically having someone ask you, 'Did you do what you said you would do?' When someone watches over you and keeps you accountable, it's much harder to give up. It's easy to fail in private when doing things on your own. Most people will easily let themselves down when no one's watching, but we don't like to let others down. This is a powerful force that we must capitalise on for success.

Accountability works best with someone you don't have a close relationship with. This is because most of us don't want to listen to a lecture from our spouse, and friends will generally let us off the hook if we give up because they don't want to feel mean. A pushy partner can cause some people to rebel and go the opposite way, just to prove a point. The best form of accountability is from someone outside your circle. Ideally someone who has a proven track record of solving the problems you are facing so they can provide the right advice when you're struggling.

Essential motivator 2: Support

It is simple to stay consistent when life is easy, but what happens when curveballs are thrown your way? For a lot of people, things start to slip. They might miss a few days' exercise, lose motivation and slip back into bad habits with food and drink. But if they can get back on track quickly, this isn't a problem.

There is always a way to work around a given situation. For example:

- Exercise can be switched or dropped altogether.

- You can compensate for doing less exercise with nutrition (such as when injured).

- Meals out at the weekend can be accounted for by eating less during the week so you can still enjoy weekends and see good results.

- Holidays can be managed if you plan ahead so you can still hit your goals long term without having to miss out on holiday fun or spend the whole time working out.

I've yet to come across an obstacle with a client that we haven't been able to find a solution for. An expert will be able to make your approach specific to you and your situation. No rigid plan or diet can do this.

When you have a coach to support you, they can see the problems before you hit them and tell you how to overcome them. You will get to your goal faster and more easily.

Essential motivator 3: Community

While having support and accountability is essential, they don't replace the power of a community. Your coach may not go through the exact same struggles as you. They may not deal with menopause symptoms or work problems or lie awake all night, unable to switch off. Nothing replaces that connection and sense of relief that can be found when you share your problems with someone who gets it.

Being part of a group of likeminded people means you can share your struggles with people who understand and work through them together, rather than feeling alone. When we see others struggle through, it gives us support to do the same. Often this can be the difference between achieving your goal and giving up early. President Kennedy said 'a rising tide lifts all boats' and this is true of being part of a community.[6] A community that succeeds as a whole will lift you up with it so you can achieve greater success.

As you work through the three stages to success – and you must work through them in order – the things you do day to day will evolve, but the three success mindsets and three essential motivators do not change. They are essential in all three phases – the reset, repetition and maintenance phases. If, once you get to your goal weight, shape and size, you get rid of the essential motivators, things will slide. Most people think they can stop once the work is done, but that isn't how it works. It is a new lifestyle and not a diet that underlies our approach. A diet gives temporary results. Lifestyle is the way you live and the success mindsets and essential motivators are key to that.

You need to follow the right process and be in the right mindset, but accountability, support and community are the backbone of every extraordinary fitness success story. They are the essence of the Fit Over 40 process and the secret that everyone who is 'effortlessly' fit and healthy uses to stay that way.

CASE STUDY: LESLEY

Lesley is a fifty-seven-year-old busy working mum with two adult children still at home. She could never stick to any diet she tried. She was caught in a vicious cycle of starting a plan, failing miserably and then feeling worse than ever. She needed an operation and wanted to be in the best possible shape to help her recovery. After 12 weeks on the programme, Lesley felt in control of food and alcohol rather than being controlled by them. She learned that it was OK to focus on herself for a while rather putting everyone else first and this helped her break that vicious cycle.

Lesley started TRINITY as a size 18 and is now wearing a size 14. She lost 10 kg (23 lbs) and almost 25 inches from all over her body and feels fantastic.

Reflection

Look back at the goals you set at the end of Chapter 1 when you answered the following question: *In a year's time, what would success look like for you?*

Then answer the questions below:

1. What is the biggest challenge to you achieving that on your own?

2. Which of the essential motivators are missing for you to turn that goal into reality? Tick all that apply:

   ☐ Accountability

   ☐ Support

   ☐ Community

Summary

There are seven success strategies that must be in place to become fit over forty and remain that way long term.

First there are the four phases of a lifetime transformation:

1. Reboot

2. Reframe

3. Reverse

4. Maintain

You must work through these in order, and each one requires a slightly different approach. The hardest is the reboot phase, which lasts 6-12 weeks, and then it gets easier.

Then there are the three essential motivators:

1. Accountability

2. Support

3. Community

These are essential to becoming fit and healthy and staying that way, regardless of age and gender. Everyone needs support, accountability and community, so that when they hit a stumbling block, they can avoid undoing all their hard work. Remove any of these and you will start slipping backwards.

PART TWO
YOUR FIT OVER 40 PROGRAMME

Now you understand the fundamental processes, mindsets and motivators needed to succeed long term, we can look at the steps to getting fit over forty. These steps will ensure that everything you do will work with your body and your hormones, rather than working against you. Your Fit Over 40 programme is the step-by-step process through which you will transform into a fit, strong, toned woman who can slip easily into your favourite clothes, set a shining example to those around you and who is bursting with energy and enthusiasm for life again.

The Fit Over 40 programme is composed of seven elements:

1. What progress to expect

2. The Diet Makeover

3. Low-impact strength training (LIST)

4. Understanding calories

5. The Stress Shield

6. Lifestyle

7. Goal-getting

We'll take each one in turn.

5

What Progress To Expect

For years, diets have conned people with unsustainable results, which leaves them disheartened because they don't get the outcome they expect. Many people love that rush of excitement that comes from stepping on the scales after a week of dieting to see it's dropped 2, 4, maybe even 6 pounds. They are convinced that this time they will succeed and that in a few weeks they'll have lost a stone.

However, this isn't always good weight loss. When you lose weight, it can come from a lot of different tissues, and it may not always be from the desirable areas. When people say they want to lose weight, what they usually mean is they want to lose fat. But diets don't measure fat loss, they measure weight loss, which is where people get conned.

This is because 60% of the body is made up of water. With simple tweaks to your diet, you can easily lose 5–10 lbs on the scales overnight. But none of this weight loss is body fat – this takes longer than a couple of days to lose. These rapid changes are always from changes in water weight and it will go straight back on once you start eating normally again.

There are two simple methods to lose water weight in a short space of time. Drop your salt intake or drop your carb intake. The more salt you eat, the more water your body will retain. If you stop eating takeaways, packaged food and ready meals, you will lose 2–5 lbs in a couple of days. But you haven't lost any fat at this point.

On top of that, for every gram of carbs you consume, your body stores 3–4 grams of water. If you stop eating carbs, not only will you have less food weight in your gut, but your body will also drop water weight as the carbs leave your system. There is nothing unhealthy about these changes in water weight, but it can be unhealthy for diets to convince you it is fat loss – this is not the case and it's not sustainable progress. Once the water weight has dropped, it will slow down.

What is unhealthy is when a diet massively cuts down how much you eat without requiring you to do any exercise. This appeals because it looks like you can lose weight without exercise. But there is a more sinister reason behind this tactic. Many diet companies don't want you to exercise. They especially want you to avoid strength training, which is the best kind of exercise for over forties, because if you don't exercise and starve your body, you will lose muscle. Losing muscle will cause your weight to fall quickly, and quicker weight loss, no matter where from, makes their diet look better.

Muscle makes you feel firm, toned, energetic and strong. It keeps your skin tight and youthful. So, while you might see record weight loss on the scales, this hides the fact that you're flabbier and weaker than ever. What's more, losing all that muscle has consequences beyond how you look. It also affects your metabolism.

Muscle is an expensive tissue for your body to maintain. Every extra bit of muscle you have burns a few more calories, even if you're doing nothing. Losing all that muscle on a diet means you will find it harder to keep the weight off afterwards as your metabolism will have slowed down and you will have to starve yourself forever to avoid the post-diet rebound.

Losing weight sustainably is a different ballgame. Losing weight over forty is another activity entirely. There are two reasons for this:

1. Muscle loss as you get older is the last thing you want. Muscle keeps you energetic, youthful, tight

and toned. It keeps your metabolism higher, so you can eat more and avoid gaining weight.

2. Weight and fat are not the same. Changes in weight can happen for a variety of reasons, and many of them have nothing to do with losing body fat.

What causes changes in weight

Lyle McDonald, in *The Women's Book*, says: 'Almost without exception, very short-term changes in scale weight tend to represent changes in water.'[7]

Five things have an impact on our water weight:

- Salt

- Carb intake

- Hydration

- Hormonal fluctuations

- Stress

We've already discussed how salt and carbohydrates can cause your body weight to go up or down. Hydration can work both ways. Drinking too much water can cause bloating, but not drinking enough can lead to water retention as your body holds onto water to survive because it doesn't know when the next drink is coming.

The impact of hormones on body weight can also be significant. During a normal monthly cycle, there are two stages where it is common to see an increase in water weight. It is normal to retain water during ovulation, about 14 days before a period starts. This may look like you've gained 2–3 lbs of fat in just a couple of days, but it is just water weight. If you are actively trying to lose fat, you may think nothing has happened despite eating well and exercising. In fact, you may have lost a pound or two of fat that week, but it is masked by an increase in water weight due to hormonal changes. This can be demotivating if you don't realise why it is happening.

Water retention can also happen in the week before a period, when oestrogen and progesterone levels rise and then fall. This can mask progress on the scales, and you may not see your weight drop even if you've been eating well and exercising regularly.

During menopause, the female sex hormones oestrogen and progesterone fluctuate unpredictably before dropping to a low level after menopause. A lot of people assume this only happens in your fifties, but for many women this can happen 5–10 years earlier. These fluctuations can again mask progress, even if you seem to be doing everything 'right'.

Lastly, stress can have an impact on the body's water balance. When stress levels are high, cortisol is elevated for sustained periods and causes water retention. This is because cortisol can bind to the same receptors that trigger water retention and, even if the bond isn't strong, there can be up to 10,000 times more cortisol in the body, making the effect pronounced.

If you have a particularly stressful week, it is common for fat loss to be masked by additional water retention. Once the stress has passed, this water weight will come off and you'll see the fruits of your labour, but you must be patient.

You should now understand why body weight is not always an accurate measure of progress, especially for women over forty. There is a better way to record your weight that takes into account these natural fluctuations which will give you the clarity to see if you are really making progress, regardless of the number on the scales each day.

How to measure progress properly

Most people are not taught the correct way to weigh themselves. They are at the mercy of whatever number appears on the scales each day, and often it's bad news.

Susan, a client of mine, weighed herself every morning or sometimes several times a day to see if her weight had changed. If the number was lower than the previous day, Susan was delighted. Sadly, those days didn't happen often. Often, Susan stepped on the scales and her weight was the same or even a pound or two higher than the day before. She almost quit but instead she decided to avoid the scales for a week. Despite giving it her all, the following week the number was the same. She assumed the diet wasn't working. That's understandable because the most common method of measuring progress is weighing yourself, and nothing changed for Susan.

Because body weight can vary day to day and even week to week, it's important to use a method of weighing that minimises the fluctuations as much as possible. I asked Susan to weigh herself every day, at the same time of day and in the same state: first thing in the morning in her underwear after using the loo.

This is important as it eradicates errors:

- Clothing can weigh a few pounds and skew your weight.

- Whether you've been to the loo or not can easily be a couple of pounds' difference on a bad day.

- It is normal to be heavier in the evening than the morning, so comparing weights from two different times of day is only going to confuse things.

The key is to weigh daily, in the same state, and take a seven-day moving average of your weight. This will flatten out any natural fluctuations and show you your 'true weight' at any point in time. There are apps available that will do this for you, such as Happy Scale on iPhone or the Libra app on Android devices. They will give you an accurate prediction of your true weight that will take some of the apprehension away from weighing yourself.

Even when weighing properly, if weight alone is the only thing you focus on, it can still be demoralising. That's why, in my programme, we use various ways to gauge progress, so that if one method does not give a clear indication of what's going on, there are other things to check. Often, even if someone's weight isn't moving that week, something else is.

The 360-degree method to measure progress

As a woman, you typically need a minimum of 20% body fat to be fit and healthy. Most people carry significantly more than this. When they lose it, they will look slimmer, leaner, more toned and ultimately feel healthier.

Therefore, you might think that we should just measure body fat itself, but measuring body fat is complicated and any affordable method is extremely inaccurate. A set of bathroom scales that measures body fat uses bio impedance analysis. When you stand on the scales, it sends an electrical current up one leg and then reads the electrical signal coming back down the other leg. It uses the change in this signal to figure out your body fat percentage. This is inaccurate for many reasons.

Firstly, often the signal passes up one leg and down the other, missing out on passing through the rest of the body. This means it is only attempting to read the body fat in your legs. Secondly, it has to distinguish between your bones, muscle, fat, organs, food, water and all the other things that make up the body, separate out the fat and then measure this on its own. People have different sized organs, muscles and bones, and the amount of food and water they retain changes day to day. A simple set of bathroom scales can't separate these things out.

You could use body fat callipers to measure skin folds instead. The theory is that you measure the same places regularly to see if the fat has reduced. However, to do it accurately you need someone else to take these measurements in precise locations on your body and it's time-consuming. It is also easy to pinch the fat harder one day than another, bringing in room for error.

The only accurate way to measure body fat is to use medical equipment, either a DEXA scanner or an MRI scanner. You'd need access to these on a regular basis and the cost takes them out of the equation for most people.

For these reasons, measuring body fat directly is not usually worth doing. You can instead measure other changes that result when body fat levels drop. When you lose body fat, your body will become smaller. Body fat is like a sponge and takes up a lot of space for its weight. By measuring different areas of the body, you can see where the fat is coming off. My clients typically measure their waist, hips, bust, legs and arms. They will often notice a change in these measurements, even if their weight hasn't shifted hugely.

Sometimes a member of my programme might be discouraged by not losing as much weight as they expected, but when they measure their body, they realise how much they have changed. Despite the scale only showing a small change, they may be able to get back into their old work trousers without having to breathe in all day. They may even go down a clothing size and rocking a new pair of jeans is far more exciting than whatever the number on the scales is saying.

It is easy to get transfixed by the number on the scales but there are a multitude of reasons why this may not change as quickly as anticipated. In the Fit Over 40 programme, we use three ways to assess our clients' progress:

1. We assess weight, using a seven-day moving average to take into account natural fluctuations

and water retention if these turn out to be problems.

2. We assess body measurements once a month to see how they are changing.

3. We get a subjective opinion on how our clients' clothes are fitting.

Often the first sign of progress is in their clothes. Their belt needs to be tightened a notch, or a pair of trousers starts to feel loose. This may be backed up by a change in measurements or in weight, but not every single week. This is normal but, provided they stay consistent and keep going, the weight and the measurements always come down in time too.

What progress to expect

We have a rule to assess what kind of progress someone can expect to see each week: the 1% rule. A person can lose up to a maximum of 1% of their body weight a week in a sustainable way. For example, someone who weighs 80 kg (about 12.5 stone) can lose 0.8 kg a week, or just under 2 lbs.

For someone heavier, they can lose more weight each week, and for someone lighter, they will not be able to lose so much sustainably. The progress you make depends on your current weight.

The 1% rule is what is possible when someone is consistent and eats the right amount for them every day, including over the weekend, and exercises three to four times a week consistently. But this may be unlikely, and it doesn't factor in hormonal changes happening over forty. It's more realistic to expect to lose 0.5–1% of your body weight per week as a woman over forty. For most women, this works out at 1–2 lbs a week. While that might not sound like much, it soon adds up.

Over 12 weeks, that's 1–2 stone in weight loss, even if you have health issues or are going through menopause. Over a year, we've seen clients lose 4–6 stone, depending on their starting weight and consistency.

The table on the following page shows what kind of weight loss is realistic depending on your starting weight.

You may be able to lose weight faster initially, even using sustainable methods such as by reducing your salt intake or carb intake, thereby reducing water retention. This will slow down after 1–2 weeks once your water levels have balanced out.

As with weight, the larger the measurement to begin with, the more it can change each month. However, it's still common for members of my programme to drop one to two dress sizes every 12 weeks.

With specific areas of the body, the biggest change is usually on the hips and waist, which can range from

Starting weight	Weight loss per week		Weight loss after 12 weeks		Weight loss after 1 year	
60 kg / 9st 6 lbs	0.3–0.6 kg	0.65–1.3 lbs	3.5–6.8 kg	8 lbs–1 st 1 lbs	13.8–24.2 kg	2 st 2 lbs–3 st 11 lbs
70 kg / 11 st	0.35–0.7 kg	0.75–1.5 lbs	4.1–8 kg	9 lbs–1 st 4 lbs	16.1–28.5 kg	2 st 7 lbs–4 st 7 lbs
80 kg / 12st 8 lbs	0.4–0.8 kg	0.9–1.75 lbs	4.7–9.1 kg	10 lbs–1 st 6 lbs	18.4–32.3 kg	2 st 13 lbs–5 st 1 lbs
90 kg / 14 st 2 lbs	0.45–0.9 kg	1–2 lbs	5.3–10.2 kg	12 lbs–1 st 8 lbs	20.7–36.6 kg	3 st 4 lbs–5 st 11 lbs
100 kg / 15 st 11lbs	0.5–1 kg	1.1–2.2 lbs	5.8–11.4 kg	13 lbs–1 st 11 lbs	23–40.7 kg	3 st 9 lbs–6 st 6 lbs
110 kg / 17 st 5lbs	0.55–1.1 kg	1.2–2.4 lbs	6.4–12.5 kg	1–2 st	25.2–44.7 kg	4 st–7st 1 lbs

1–2 inches per month, whereas smaller areas of the body, such as the legs and arms, often change less. However, everyone's body is different, and everyone has stubborn areas of fat.

Stubborn areas of body fat

Stubborn areas are slower to change initially than others. This could be your stomach, limbs or lower half – your bum and legs. Stubborn areas tend to hold onto fat for longer. It can take over 12 weeks for some areas to change, while the weight practically falls off other areas in the first few weeks.

Where your stubborn areas are depends primarily on your genetics and hormone balance, and it can shift depending on your lifestyle and different life stages. It is common around the menopause to develop 'middle-aged spread'. This is because oestrogen and progesterone drop, while testosterone levels remain roughly the same. Because testosterone levels become higher compared to oestrogen and progesterone, this causes more fat to be stored around the middle rather than on the legs and bum.

However, you don't need to despair about your stubborn areas of body fat. As long as you have the right approach and are consistent, the excess fat can and will be lost even from stubborn areas.

CASE STUDY: CAROLINE

Several years ago, I worked with Caroline, a mum of two teenagers who worked full-time as a manager in a stressful job in Oxfordshire. Caroline is a great example of the 1% rule. She started off at 15 st 6 lbs (97.8 kg). Size 14s no longer fitted her comfortably, but she refused to buy a size 16. She regularly did spinning classes and also lifted weights in the gym on her own, but nothing she did got the weight moving.

On my programme, Caroline lost 4.5 stone (26.4 kg) and got down to wearing size 12s comfortably, even size 10s in certain clothes. She even wore a bikini on holiday for the first time in as long as she could remember.

This change didn't happen overnight. She lost that 4.5 stone over a year, which averages out at exactly 1 lb a week. Losing 1–2 lbs a week might not sound exciting, but it's sustainable and adds up quickly. Caroline transformed her diet, exercise and mindset. We have stayed in touch since we finished working together, and because she lost the weight in a sustainable way, while learning exactly how she had done it, she was able to maintain her new strong, lean and toned figure, whereas previously she'd always fallen off the wagon and regained the weight within months.

Reflection

Here's how to work out what kind of weight loss is sustainable for you using the 1% rule. There are three steps to follow:

- Take your current body weight either in pounds or kilograms (it's more complex in stone, so avoid that here).

- Multiply that number by 0.005. That will give you the lower end of what's possible for you each week.

- Now multiply your body weight by 0.01. That will give you the top end of what's possible for you each week.

You can note that down below for reference.

Sustainable weight loss for me is between ___ and ___ each week.

Summary

It's important to have realistic expectations of what you can achieve when losing weight as a woman over forty. The 1% rule means a person can lose 0.5–1% of their body weight per week sustainably, and this is the best way to assess whether you're making good progress.

It's important to measure progress in a number of ways, and not just by weighing yourself, as there are many reasons why your body weight may not drop, even if you've done everything right.

I recommend using a combination of body weight (ideally using an app to take a seven-day moving average), body measurements and judging how you feel in your clothes to assess your progress as accurately as possible.

6

The Diet Makeover

If you don't get your nutrition right, you will not lose weight even if you have a holistic approach which includes exercise and mindset. No amount of exercise or positive thinking will shift the fat, especially as you get older. You can't out-exercise the wrong diet. You *must* get your nutrition right to see results.

I have helped over 5,000 women succeed with the nutrition strategies in this book. They still eat with the family, enjoy socialising with friends and can even have their favourite foods along with a few drinks and see good results.

But how do they achieve that? It starts with a process we call the Diet Makeover.

A Diet Reset

People know they should eat a 'balanced diet' – not too many processed foods, cook from scratch and avoid takeaways, sugar, fizzy drinks and alcohol. While they may not be sure what exactly they should be doing, most people know what they *shouldn't* be doing. Yet they can't seem to stop doing it.

That's where the Diet Makeover comes in. It's a reset that enables you to find that 'balanced diet' as quickly as possible. It reignites your energy levels and unlocks mental clarity so that you feel alert, focused and alive. You can also lose up to 10 lbs in 2 weeks without doing anything dangerous or drastic.

Most people try to gradually improve their diet. They try to eat less sugar, reduce alcohol and cut back on treats. But one biscuit or 'just one drink' adds up over the week and can become a whole packet of biscuits and a whole bottle of wine, which is the equivalent of eating thirteen chicken breasts or ten medium baked potatoes extra that week.

If you've tried to eat or drink less, you know how hard this is. The problem is that the habits and cravings are deeply ingrained. One stressful day at work and the treats, takeaways and wine become too tempting.

The Diet Makeover fixes all that. It resets your cravings and habits with food and drink. It clears the slate and many of our clients report their cravings have totally vanished and their energy is through the roof within 1–2 weeks. You simply need to cut out four problem food groups that cause the most cravings, bad habits and ultimately weight gain.

These are what we call the WADS foods:

- Wheat

- Alcohol

- Dairy

- Sugar

These food groups are chosen for three reasons:

1. They are all high in calories, which makes them easy to over-consume and gain weight (or prevent weight loss). By cutting them out, you will quickly and easily start to lose weight.

2. People crave sugar and alcohol, and the more you consume, the worse the cravings get. The only way to eliminate the cravings is to go 'cold turkey' for a short period of time.

3. People can have issues with digesting wheat and/ or dairy. This can lead to severe bloating, which can mask any fat loss progress, as well as cause energy levels to plummet, skin to break out and a number of other issues. The quickest and easiest way to know if they cause you any issues is to cut

them out and then reintroduce them one at a time. This is cheaper and more reliable than much of the 'intolerance testing' available.

The Diet Makeover will kickstart your weight loss and send your energy levels skywards, but there's one thing you must complete first to ensure it goes smoothly, otherwise you will fall at the first hurdle. We call this the Cupboard Cleanse.

The Cupboard Cleanse

Before you start eating better, you need to set yourself up to succeed. Most people fail with any change in diet because they convince themselves they can rely on willpower. The willpower delusion is a trap many fall into when trying to achieve anything new. They believe willpower is needed for success, and that it's something you can get more of. This is wrong.

Willpower doesn't work because it is a finite resource. Just like your phone, the more you use it, the more you drain your battery until it runs out and stops working. The same is true of willpower due to something called decision fatigue. This is the theory that you only have a finite amount of decision-making ability each day; with every decision you make, the less willpower you have left. After a busy week at work and at home, most people burn through their willpower reserves quickly. By the end of the week, willpower has gone.

They turn to wine, crisps or chocolate and, because these foods are so high in calories, they quickly undo any hard work eating well and exercising.

If you want to succeed, you need to eliminate willpower from the equation and use something that is reliable. That means changing your environment, which is a much more reliable predictor of results than willpower. Making changes to your environment makes it easier to do what's right without having to think about staying motivated. If you set up your surroundings so that making the best decisions comes easily, you will find it easier to practise better habits. If you change your environment, you change your results.

Disciplined people have no more willpower than anyone else when put into tempting situations. They appear disciplined because they structure their lives so that they avoid tempting situations in the first place and rarely need to use willpower.

Success, therefore, is nothing to do with willpower and everything to do with making your environment work for you. How do you do this? With nutrition, it needs to be easy to make healthy food choices and difficult to make unhealthy food choices. The simplest rule is that if it's not in your house, you can't consume it.

Members of my programmes implement the Cupboard Cleanse by removing the processed treats, snacks, comfort food and alcohol from their cupboards and replacing them with better alternatives. This is then followed by the Diet Makeover, removing anything containing the WADS foods – wheat, alcohol, dairy and sugar – for 1-2 weeks.

Many people find it hard to throw food away, but if you eat it you will gain even more fat and be on the back foot before you start. You can always give the food away to a local food bank or to friends and family. If you can't give the food away or bin it, make the food hard to access. Out of sight, out of mind.

Here are some strategies that work well for women on my programmes:

- Put alcohol in the garage in a box. Place that box beneath several others so it is hard to access. You will have to plan to have a drink rather than it being readily available to sabotage your progress after a stressful day.

- If you must have treats in the cupboard for your children, buy them the treats you like the least. Move snacks to the back of a different cupboard to where you used to keep them. This breaks the pattern of looking in the usual places when bored.

- Get a food lock box. Many of my clients' children love using them to keep their treats safe from their parents. Your children or your partner sets the code so only they can access it.

You must make good habits easy and bad habits difficult if you want to succeed. Skip this step and you will fail.

Once you have cleansed your cupboards, it's time to restock with lots of tasty healthy foods. For the Diet Makeover, this is anything that doesn't contain the WADS foods. Focus on eating single-ingredient foods such as lean meat and fish, whole fruit and vegetables and lots of grains and pulses. Note that fruit sugars found in whole unprocessed fruit are not the same as processed sugar. That means you can eat as much fruit as you like.

We recommend doing the Diet Makeover for 1–2 weeks, and then you can move onto the next step, which is more flexible and sustainable long term. You must reset everything first so that you start from a solid foundation. Keep it simple and don't worry if you repeat some of your meals and snacks – it's easier that way. Eating the same breakfast and lunch every day keeps things quick and easy, then dinners can be tailored to suit your family's needs.

The Diet Makeover will reset your cravings, get you into good habits and ensure you're eating the right kind of foods that will work with your changing hormones, while avoiding those that will work against them.

CASE STUDY: SARAH

Sarah, forty-four and a mother of two, worked full-time in the insurance industry. She used the Diet Makeover to transform her relationship with alcohol. Sarah went from drinking almost every evening, which had caused her weight to spiral out of control, to losing weight and no longer thinking about alcohol at all!

Despite an active lifestyle, Sarah had ended up relying on alcohol and food for comfort. She didn't really enjoy life and dealt with that by drinking every night, which resulted in not feeling great the next day. Then her stepfather was diagnosed with lymphoma and she realised she needed to stop drinking in order to support her family properly. Not only that, she realised her drinking had affected her job and was making her overweight. She'd tried Weight Watchers, the Dukan Diet and the GI diet, which worked short-term, but she could never keep them up and the weight always piled back on again afterwards.

Sarah joined my programme and went from a size 16 to a size 8. She now says: 'I feel comfortable in my skin, I love my body. I feel strong and fit!'

The Diet Makeover helped Sarah to reset unhealthy habits and transform not only her body but her whole life. She got control over her drinking. 'I feel really healthy,' she says. 'I feel really strong. I love that I can do press-ups. I go to bed at a decent time now. I sleep well.' She feels that she has transformed into 'somebody who owns who I am. I love who I am. I have taken ownership of my life.'

Whether you drink regularly, can't control your sugar cravings or consume too many lattés, the Diet Makeover will eliminate the cravings, get the scales moving and get you into a healthy balanced diet as quickly as possible.

Reflection

Complete your own Diet Makeover at home for 1–2 weeks and see how much better you feel for it. Try getting your family involved to help with accountability.

You can download a Diet Makeover-friendly shopping list, cookbook and survival guide for free at trinitytransformation.co.uk/dietmakeover.

Summary

You must get your nutrition right to lose weight – you can't out-exercise the wrong diet. However, if you've got strong cravings and are stuck in bad habits with alcohol or comfort foods, a hard reset is the only way to get back to a healthy balanced diet.

The Diet Makeover is a 1–2 week reset that involves eliminating the four biggest 'problem foods' in the western diet:

- Wheat
- Alcohol
- Dairy
- Sugar

There are two stages to the Diet Makeover:

1. The Cupboard Cleanse
2. The Diet Makeover itself

The Cupboard Cleanse involves setting up your environment for success by clearing your cupboards of tempting comfort foods, so you don't have to rely on willpower to succeed (which never works if you have a stressful day-to-day life).

The Diet Makeover then involves cutting out the WADS foods and replacing them with healthy filling alternatives that will boost your energy and get the scales moving in the right direction.

7

Low-Impact
Strength Training

Traditional diets take one of two stances with exercise. One focuses on cardio in the belief that it burns most fat. The other focuses on drastically restricting your diet but with no exercise. Neither work well if you want to get fit over forty.

Fad diets advocate no exercise because they know humans are inherently lazy. It is far easier to sell someone weight loss with no exercise whatsoever than tell them they have to work out multiple times a week, every week, for months. But this isn't done just to make it easy – they have an ulterior motive. A fad diet would rather you did no exercise at all because the goal is not to get you fit and healthy but to lose as much weight as possible so they can lure you in and make a big profit.

By starving your body and avoiding exercise, you will lose a lot of muscle, which will look great on the scales, but won't look so good in the mirror. This also impacts your metabolism. The more muscle someone has, the more calories they will burn just by being alive. After a fad diet, the opposite happens. They have less muscle, which means their metabolism slows down. It creates a vicious cycle of having to eat less just to keep the weight off, let alone to lose any more.

Avoiding exercise is also not good for your mental health and energy levels. A review of the research on exercise and mental health reported that 'exercise improves mental health by reducing anxiety, depression, and negative mood and by improving self-esteem and cognitive function'.[8]

Exercise makes us feel good. It makes us feel human. It makes us feel tired in the evening so we can get a proper night's sleep and perform at our best every day. If we stop exercising, we lose these benefits.

Many women choose the wrong kind of exercise to get fit over forty, making it more difficult for themselves, and become discouraged. For example, they think that sweaty cardio in a gym class or running is the only way to get the weight off. But these won't get you far if you want to get fit over forty.

The cardio trap

Cardio exercise is anything that gets the heart racing. There are two key types of cardio, each with their own pitfalls.

LISS

Low-impact steady state exercises are those where you do the same thing at the same pace for a long period of time, such as running, jogging, swimming or cycling. Your heart rate will increase and it will be a bit harder to breathe, but you should be able to keep going for 20–30 minutes or longer.

The main benefit of LISS is that it improves your cardiovascular fitness, which is good for your heart health. However, it is not great for changing your figure or getting lean and toned over forty. As women get older, their bodies naturally start to lose muscle. To burn enough calories for it to be worth doing, LISS training generally needs to be done for 30–40 minutes as a minimum. However, once you start doing cardio for over half an hour or so, your body starts to burn muscle for energy. This is the muscle that makes you strong, firm and toned. Having more muscle also gives you a faster metabolism. By doing steady state cardio, you actually make it harder to be firm and toned as you burn your precious muscle. It also makes it harder to keep the weight off over time as your metabolism will slow down the more muscle you lose.

Unless you absolutely love this kind of exercise, it is best avoided if you want to be fit over forty, as it is not time efficient and can slow the process down.

HIIT

High-intensity interval training alternates between exercises that are high intensity, such as jumping up and down onto a high box, with exercises that are relatively low intensity, for example, resting completely or pedalling an exercise bike on a low gear for 20–30 seconds. HIIT can burn a lot of calories in a short time and works well for young people, who are already fit and have low body fat levels. These, funnily enough, are the people who usually appear in the marketing videos for HIIT training.

However, HIIT training can put a huge strain on your body. It will spike the stress hormone cortisol. As you now know, it is key to keep cortisol under control to lose weight quickly and easily over forty, especially if your life is stressful. Therefore HIIT training can actually make it harder to lose weight for women over forty!

Injury risk is also high with HIIT training, because excess body fat puts strain on the joints when jumping up and down, and the older someone gets, the less their joints will tolerate this. It can eventually lead to bad backs, knees or sore shoulders and worse. The good news that is you don't need to do any cardio to get fit over forty.

The best exercise for women over forty

There are many exercises you can do over forty – yoga, Pilates, running, cycling, going to the gym or swimming. But some forms of exercise produce better physical results than others and are easier to keep up. The key is the difference between *exercise* and *training*.

Exercise is when someone picks something with little thought or understanding of whether it will bring them the result they want. This means that, when they exercise, it's a struggle and the results are poor. They do it because they feel they have to, not because they want to.

Training is methodical, structured and, most importantly, is designed to achieve progress towards a goal. Training makes your dream a reality. The truth is that no one really wants to exercise. They want the results of exercise, to look and feel better, but they don't know how.

Over forty, the changes in your physiology and hormones mean that only specific types of exercise will shift the weight and tone you up. You are now fighting a battle on four frontiers:

- Stress

- Joint degradation

- Muscle loss

- Time

The female body becomes more sensitive to stress with age, making weight loss difficult over forty. It is important to choose exercise that doesn't add too much additional stress. This rules out HIIT, hard spinning sessions, burpees or brutal circuits. High impact exercise like running or jumping up and down should also be avoided because it places additional wear and tear on the joints, and the more excess weight you carry, the bigger the strain on your joints.

When jogging, your foot striking the ground creates an impact force of three to four times your body weight. For the average client, weighing 12 stone (around 76 kg), this means their leg joints will be subject to almost 50 stone or 300 kg – the equivalent of walking around with a grand piano on your back.

However, not all force through the joints is bad. *Appropriate* force through your bones and joints is important, especially for women over forty. This is because women are more prone to osteoporosis as they get older, which is when bones become porous and weaken over time. If you sit down all day, your body will not get the signals it needs to prioritise and maintain bone density, and this can lead to osteoporosis.

Carefully applying appropriate loads to your body will signal the need to increase bone density, and the easiest way to do this is through the right kind of exercise. This force must be carefully controlled to avoid injury or damage to the joints, especially for anyone carrying extra weight.

The best way to achieve these things is through strength training, specifically through low-impact strength training (LIST). This means lifting weights in a slow and controlled way. The benefit of this is that it still burns calories effectively, just like cardio, but it keeps stress levels low. Neither does it require loads of equipment. You just need two to three weights and a resistance band and you're good to go.

It is also time efficient. You can achieve great results in a short space of time compared to cardio. My clients typically do just three workouts a week for 30–45 minutes a time (including a full warm-up). Most clients do this from home so they can fit their workouts into their schedule easily without taking much time away from work or family life.

Finally, it builds muscle, which is the opposite of most cardio exercise. Not only will this muscle make you feel firm, toned, energetic and youthful, it also has another little-known benefit. Building muscle is an investment in your metabolism.

To maintain your figure, you must keep doing the same amount of cardio exercise. What's more, over time the cardio exercise will burn your muscle for energy, especially as you get older and muscle becomes harder to maintain. The amount of muscle you have affects your metabolism, so losing muscle means you need to *increase* the amount of cardio you're doing over the years just to maintain your figure, let alone to change and improve it.

LIST, however, is an investment in your body. Each time you work out, you signal to your muscles to come back stronger and more toned. As you build muscle, your metabolism increases, which means you can eat more and maintain your weight. Or if you do build more muscle, you could eat the same amount that previously meant you maintained your weight and you'd now lose weight. Either way, it's a win-win. You feel firm and toned from LIST and find it easier to lose weight and keep it off.

Some women worry that strength training will make them big and bulky. This may be because of images of female bodybuilders. They worry the same will happen to them if they lift weights. This won't happen because bodybuilders train hard with weights for decades and meticulously control their diet. They may also use performance-enhancing drugs like steroids, meaning their testosterone levels are artificially elevated, resulting in far more muscle than you will ever have naturally.

Typically, my clients become smaller, slimmer and more toned, all from strength training. It is by far the best way to get fit over forty and prevent many of the side effects of ageing.

If you're new to strength training, I'd recommend starting with two to three workouts a week for 30–45 minutes. That should be plenty to get the weight moving.

Once you've started doing LIST consistently for a week or so, it's time to move onto the next stage with your nutrition.

CASE STUDY: SARAH

Sarah, who we met in the previous chapter, was sceptical about not doing any cardio and trying a new type of exercise. She thought cardio was essential to lose weight. However, on my programme she lost a lot of weight without doing any cardio. When she started, Sarah was 11 stone 3 pounds (71.5 kg). Now she is 8 stone (50.8 kg). Her friends thought it was through running. When she told them she wasn't running, they didn't believe her. 'It's like people don't want to hear that because they believe it's something else,' she said. 'The strength training, balancing out my food and all the other stuff is how I lost the weight. Any cardio is just a bit of an added extra for me now and I do it for my own mindset because I love going out for a run with a friend – that's my fun time now.'

Reflection

Want to try out a LIST workout? You can try out three free on-demand LIST workouts at www.trinitytransformation.co.uk/workouts.

All you'll need is a resistance band, which can be found for under £10, or kettlebells or dumbbells, which can be sourced for under £50. I've provided links to both at the web address above along with the workouts, so you can get started today and begin to reap the benefits.

Summary

It's important to choose the right kind of exercise when trying to get fit over forty. While in your twenties and thirties you may have been able to get away with almost anything and see progress, you now need something that works with your changing body or it will be difficult to progress at all.

This needs a programme that:

- Keeps stress levels low
- Is gentle on joints
- Keeps metabolism high
- Maintains bone density

Many popular forms of exercise, such as long-distance cardio, HIIT and gym classes, make these things worse, not better, making it much harder to lose weight than it needs to be.

Members of my programme follow an exercise methodology called LIST. They do just three to four workouts a week for 30–45 minutes (including a full warm-up) and they are typically able to lose 1–2 stone every 12 weeks, working out at home.

8
Understanding Calories

The science is simple. If you consume too many calories, you will gain weight.

However, just because the science is simple, following it isn't always easy. Many things can make it easy for people to consume too many calories. For example, unmanaged stress, hormonal changes, bad habits, social pressure and simply not understanding where hidden calories lie in food and drink.

A calorie is a way of measuring the energy contained in food and drink. If our body has more energy coming in than it can use, it has no choice but to store the rest as body fat. If it has less energy coming in than it needs, known as a calorie deficit, it has to come up with the energy from elsewhere by breaking down muscle or body fat.

This last distinction is important. It is possible on starvation diets to lose lots of weight, but much of that comes from muscle, which will leave you feeling weak and flabby, not toned and energetic. This is because they reduce calories too much, along with cutting out strength-based exercise, which leaves the body with no choice but to burn muscle for energy.

How many calories should you consume to lose weight?

There is no magic calorie number. Some fad diets claim 800 calories or 1,200 calories is best, but both of these are too low to be healthy for most people and will lead to muscle loss, as well as poor energy levels. Diets like these have poor adherence because they are so restrictive.

There is a sweet spot in terms of calories which works best for each person, where they have enough calories to make it sustainable so they can still enjoy a varied diet and have a social life, but not too many calories, so that their body still has to burn some body fat for energy.

A person's calorie target should take into account their age, height, weight, body fat percentage, body fat distribution, dieting history and any health conditions. It should also factor in things like menopause, PCOS and thyroid conditions. This target should also incorporate your current activity levels. If you sit at a desk all day, you will need to eat less than someone who walks 15,000 steps a day.

You can get an estimate of what this number is for you using my Fit Over 40 calorie calculator at www.trinitytransformation.co.uk/calculator.

In my programmes, we work this out for our clients individually. It can be trial and error at first to find that sweet spot, but once we have it right, it is not unusual for our clients to lose 1–2 stone in just 12 weeks. We'll discuss how to use this calorie number shortly, but first it's important to understand why diets often avoid the C-word, and why you shouldn't.

Why diets avoid the C-word

Most diets don't discuss calories. If they can convince you they have a special points system, or a special nutritional approach, you are stuck with them because you don't know how to manage your nutrition and lose weight any other way.

In reality, all diets are based on calories. The only way you can lose weight is to consume fewer calories than your body needs each day, which forces it to burn fat (or muscle) to get the extra energy it needs to survive. All diets work this way, whether or not they tell you this. A points system is simply a way of listing the calories in food, an unnecessary step to make you think they have a magic system. They may also avoid teaching you to read normal food labels so you end up buying their branded diet food, resulting in more profit for them.

Low carb is another fad diet that is thought to work due to some special science. People think carbs are fattening. But carbs are not fattening on their own. Consuming too many calories is fattening. If you cut out an *entire* food group like carbs, you cut out about 60% of the calories in the average person's diet – no wonder they lose weight. It's not magic, it's simply cutting calories, but for many people it's not sustainable.

Fasting is another diet that claims to be special, on which you are only allowed to eat for a few hours a day. Funnily enough, doing this means you will eat less than if you ate all day long. It does not have any special fat burning mechanism, it's simply a way of reducing your calorie intake.

Why diets don't work

Firstly, diets have loopholes. With a low carb diet, you can eat as many high fat foods as you like. This dietary fat doesn't automatically make you fat. But if you consume too many calories, even if you're not eating carbs, you won't lose weight. This is easily done because dietary fat is more calorie-dense than the other two key macronutrients, carbohydrates and protein.

Dietary fat has nine calories per gram, whereas carbohydrates and protein contain just four calories per gram. Often foods such as nuts, avocado and dark chocolate, as well as fattier cuts of meat and fish like steak and salmon, are recommended on a low carb diet but they actually contain lots of calories so it's possible to eat too much without realising.

A points system can also be exploited. They allow free foods such as unlimited pasta or avocados. This free rein means people can make slow progress, if any at all, because they are still able to eat far too many calories within the rules.

Secondly, most diets are not optimised for over forties. They don't account for changing hormones, or how the stress hormone response changes with age, especially for women. If they provide you with calorie targets, they often only base them on a couple of factors such as your starting body weight and activity level, but this will not cut it over forty for all the reasons we've discussed.

Thirdly, most diets are not sustainable. The golden rule of sustainability is that if you can't follow it long term, the results will only ever be temporary. Most diets require drastic changes and don't fit around people's normal lives, meaning people only stick to them for a few weeks or months at a time. They may see some progress, but if they can't stick to it, they go back to their old habits, and their body goes back to how it was before.

To lose weight and keep it off, it's important to do something that is sustainable, flexible and fits around your life, so you can keep it up long term.

The sustainable way to track calories

Tracking calories is the *only* way to guarantee you lose weight. It's like managing your finances. Your calories are your budget for the day. 'Spend' too much and you will go into debt. This debt means gaining body fat. But if you don't spend everything, you will benefit from that in the future. Over time, keeping to your calorie budget will result in steady sustainable weight loss.

The big benefit of tracking calories is that it's flexible. You don't need to ban anything. You can still eat with your family, grab food on the go, eat out and have a treat or a few drinks, provided you make it work within your calorie 'budget'.

These days, it couldn't be easier to do. You can simply download a phone app that's designed for the job. This app will remember your favourite foods, store your recipes, scan the barcodes of almost all packaged foods and even contains most of the food found in major restaurants.

Paul Mort, a former mentor of mine and Master Coach of the Year 2020, says: 'If someone can't be bothered to spend five minutes a day putting what they eat into their phone, they don't deserve to lose weight.'[9] Most people who avoid tracking their calories do so because they don't want to face the truth – that they are not losing weight because they eat and drink too much. When you accept this, it will liberate you, stop you relying unsustainable diets and allow you to start seeing results.

Common calorie tracking mistakes

Many people make mistakes when tracking calories that means it won't work at all. These are some common traps.

Not measuring properly

The difference between losing weight sustainably and maintaining a steady weight is only about 15–20% in terms of your calorie intake. Consequently, it only takes a few small errors in tracking to make the difference between maintaining and losing weight. Therefore it's important to measure out anything you eat or drink as accurately as possible.

This doesn't apply to pre-made food in packets, where you can scan the barcode. Nor does it apply to eating out at restaurants, but it does apply to anything you make from scratch at home, or you measure out yourself (such as alcohol).

You'll need a good set of food scales and a measuring jug for this. A shot measurer is essential if you drink spirits, as it's all too easy for a 'small' gin to actually be a triple, and it only takes two of those to completely undo your calorie deficit. Get in the habit of measuring food and drink before you consume it at home, ideally in its uncooked state.

Tracking apps allow you enter cooked food, but this is less accurate as the amount of water the food will absorb or lose in cooking will vary depending on how it is cooked. It's not the end of the world if you weigh things cooked – it's still more accurate than not weighing it at all, and usually still works well enough.

You may not be able to weigh absolutely everything you eat. If a friend has cooked for you, search for that meal in your tracking app and it will usually have some ready meal variation. It's not perfect, but it's unlikely to happen that often and it will still be much better than not tracking it at all.

The most important thing is to weigh or measure things whenever you can. If you do that, you will see fast progress, and that will keep you motivated to keep tracking and get that weight off.

Tracking in retrospect

One of the most common calorie tracking mistakes is tracking in retrospect. That's because it is too easy to forget exactly what you've eaten, whether on purpose or by accident. Research by the UK's Behavioural Insights Team found that Britons under-reported their food intake by 50% on average – they didn't account for *half* of what they had eaten, because they forgot or estimated the quantities to be far less than the reality.[10]

If you don't track as you go, you can't tweak what you are eating and make it work for you. If you track it before you've eaten, you'll be able to see how many calories you've got left for the day and make sure that choice is right for you. You can scan a product and know immediately if you have enough calories left in your day to allow you to eat it and still see results, or if you need to pick something else.

This is the best way to educate yourself on what's a good choice for you and what's not – but *only* if you track in advance of eating or drinking it.

Weekends

People can fall down with calorie tracking at the week-ends, even after being consistent all week. They have a glass of wine after a stressful week and maybe they track it. Before they know it, the whole bottle is gone. They tell themselves they will enter it into the app later. However, often they forget, spend the next day eating to ease their hangover and don't track anything else until Monday. It's only when you track a weekend in full you become aware of how much you have eaten.

The average Indian takeaway is around 1,300 calo-ries, which is more than 80% of the daily calorie target I give my average client. A pack of biscuits, a large sharing bag of crisps or a couple of bottles of wine is roughly the same in terms of calorie content. These things can seem relatively innocent on their own, but decisions like that over the weekend will put the brakes on your weight loss.

The only way to really know if what you are eating and drinking is working for you is to track *your whole week* and learn how these foods stack up. It only takes 5 minutes a day to track your calories properly and it will guarantee you see results.

Using the app's calorie and nutrition targets

Most calorie tracking apps will give you an estimate of how many calories you should consume to hit your weight loss goals. However, they often generate these numbers from very little data, which means they can be inaccurate. Often, I give a client a target that is 500 calories different to what an app has given them. I take into account complications such as menopausal changes, thyroid issues and their dieting history to give them a calorie target that will work well for them and be sustainable.

My team have perfected this process for the women we work with. We have created a calculator that can help with your calorie targets if you're unsure where to start. You can access this at www.trinitytransforma-tion.co.uk/calculator.

Remember, this is still only an estimate, and it can take a bit of tweaking to find the right amount for you. I calculate a 'best guess' for my clients based on the information collected during our initial assessments, and then after 2 weeks we analyse their real-world process and make changes to get the best possible results.

It's not uncommon for clients to tell me they think the number I've given them is too high initially, only for them to lose half a stone within the first few weeks and report it's the first time they've lost that much weight so quickly without being starving all the time.

Aiming too low

Many people think they have to starve themselves to lose weight. A lot of diets will give you 1,200 calories or fewer, which is too generic and too low for most women. However, many still don't lose weight despite this low calorie target. There are a few reasons this can happen.

First of all, people on very low calories can get stuck in a starvation-binge cycle. This means they stick to their diet for a few days, but it's a real struggle as they're hungry all the time. Eventually they can't keep it up any longer and they spend a few days 'off the wagon', ordering takeaways, drinking regularly, eating comfort food and having whatever they like. This never works.

The most important driver of results is your calorie average *over the week*. For someone stuck in the starvation-binge cycle, they eat as many calories as they normally would over the course of the week, they just eat a lot less at the beginning of the week and a lot more at the end of the week. This means they cannot lose weight, as their weekly calorie average is still too high.

Another way people deal with starvation diets is not tracking everything they consume properly. They don't measure correctly. They underestimate what they eat. They don't include calories in cooking oil or alcohol, and they might skip the latté they picked up on the way to work. As a result, instead of eating 1,200 calories, they actually eat 1,800 or 2,000 calories a day, but their app still says 1,200 calories. They blame calorie tracking, when in fact it was the unsustainably low number of calories that doomed them from the outset.

The best approach is to aim for a realistic number of calories. Something low enough to lose weight consistently at the maximum sustainable rate (remember the 1% rule), but not so low that it is difficult to stick to.

Many clients tell me that what they're doing doesn't feel hard – it doesn't feel like a diet to them, so they can stick to it consistently for months, which is important as often that's how long it takes to significantly change your body for the better.

Managing calories long term

Anything you can't keep up long term will only ever give temporary results. This is true of calorie tracking too, but you don't need to track calories forever. Calorie tracking is an exception to this rule, because by losing weight through tracking you will learn what is in different types of food and drink, what will work for you and what won't, and how to assess new things that you have not come across before so they don't catch you out. Once you've learned this, you will be equipped with the tools you need to stay fit over forty for the rest of your life.

Maintaining your weight is not as difficult as losing weight. My clients often keep the excess weight off with ease without having to track everything they consume, where previously it would pile back on within months of finishing a diet. However, this relies on several other factors.

Stress can directly and indirectly stop progress in its tracks. If you don't manage it properly, knowing your calorie target is worthless as you won't be able to stick to it.

That's what led us to develop our Stress Shield process, which means our clients are able to see good results no matter what life throws at them.

CASE STUDY: JULIE

When Julie joined my programme, she was bursting out of her size 16s. Her loft was full of clothes that hadn't fitted for years. She lived in stretchy clothes because they were the only thing that was comfortable. She'd tried a number of diets, but she found them restrictive and could never keep them up long term. She also did spinning classes five times a week but never noticed any difference in how she looked or felt.

During the programme, Julie learned how to track calories *the right way* without feeling like she was on a diet. She thought she'd find tracking calories difficult before she started the programme, especially since she works as a busy social worker, so she worried she wouldn't have time. But she found it easy when done our way, and now it's second nature. She eats the same meals as her family, and just makes sure the portion sizes work for her. As a result, she lost 2 stone (13 kg) and got down to the lightest weight she'd been in 35 years, all in under 6 months.

Reflection

The number of calories you need to consume to lose weight sustainably will be unique to you. You can get an estimate of what this number is for you using my Fit Over 40 calorie calculator at www.trinitytransformation.co.uk/calculator.

Summary

To lose weight, you must consume fewer calories than your body burns each day. This is how all diets work, even if they hide it behind a points system or fancy explanation.

If you want to lose weight, you must consume the right number of calories for you. This will be unique to you and must take into account your age, weight, body fat percentage, activity levels and any health conditions.

You can use a smartphone app to track your calorie intake, and it can be done quickly and easily. Tracking calories is more flexible than any other weight loss approach, as you get to choose how you 'spend' your calorie budget, and it's easy to fit in a few treats as long as you don't go overboard.

9
The Stress Shield

Stress can have a serious impact on getting fit over forty. It directly affects weight loss by changing your hormones, which can make weight loss harder. But stress also indirectly affects weight loss by taking your focus away from your health and fitness goals. When people get stressed, they go back to their old habits – skipping exercise, drinking too much, comfort eating or ordering takeaways. Turning to food and drink is not a productive way to manage your stress levels. Poorly managed stress is one of the main reasons so many people struggle to lose weight over forty.

Life is stressful. The older you get, the more responsibility you're likely to have at home and at work. But you have a choice. You can either proactively manage that stress through things you *choose* to do, or you can manage it subconsciously through coping mechanisms like food and drink. In her book, *Why Good People Do Bad Things*, Debbie Ford compares unmanaged emotions to trying to hold a beach ball underwater. Initially, you can do it and no one can see it's there. But it only takes one little thing to knock it off balance. When that happens, the ball breaks free and bursts through the surface, spraying water every-where and making a mess.[11]

The same happens with stress. If you suppress it for too long, eventually the pressure will get too much and must be released, often in undesirable ways like eating and drinking. Ignoring stress and 'powering through' is not a strategy. It might mean the work gets done or the family get what they need, but your own health and happiness will get sacrificed in the pro-cess. You need to let that stress out so that the pressure doesn't rise to breaking point, when good intentions go out of the window.

My clients use a process we've developed called the Stress Shield that takes less than 10 minutes a day to bring stress levels down, and over time it builds up mental resilience so they don't turn to food and drink even when life throws them a curveball.

Part 1: Meditation

What happens when you have a stressful situation at work or at home? For most people, they dive headfirst into solving it, often at the expense of everything else.

Let's call the situation that happened 'the event', and the thing you do as a result of it 'the reaction'. For a lot of people, this reaction becomes instant. It has been done so many times that it now happens automatically. This is called automaticity, and it's why so many people end up on the sofa with a glass of wine or a pack of chocolate without knowing quite how they got there.

Automaticity can be useful. Like those moments when you realise you've driven the last five miles without thinking. But it can also be dangerous; if you get too caught up in everything, you can't take a step back to think if this is really the best decision for you in the long run. If that's the case, then you'll forever find yourself sabotaging your best efforts to get fit over forty.

The quality of your life comes down to the quality of all the seemingly insignificant decisions you make on a daily basis, all added up together. If you want to get a different result, a better result, whether that's with your health and fitness or elsewhere in your life, you need to make different decisions.

To do this, you have to create the headspace and the clarity to make those decisions. As a mentor of mine once put it, 'you need to stop running round like a fire-fighting hero' fixing irrelevant problems, while losing sight of the most important things – you and your goals.

Meditation will do all that for you. It has the added benefit of reducing cortisol levels, which makes fat loss much easier to achieve for women over forty who naturally have a heightened stress response due to their age.

There are many forms of meditation available through free apps, making it easy to find one that suits you. My favourite meditation app is Insight Timer, which is free at the time of writing. You can search for what you're struggling with that day and get a guided meditation specifically to help with that challenge. I recommend starting small. When my clients first start doing their daily Stress Shield, they start with just 2 minutes of meditation a day and they still feel the benefits.

People think meditation is about 'not thinking' or 'clearing your mind' but my meditation teacher, Arjuna Ishaya, taught me that thoughts during meditation are simply stress being released, and the more stressed you are, the more thoughts you'll have.

Meditation can seem like a strange concept for us success-driven westerners. We want to do it 'right'. But it's important to surrender to the process and see what it brings each day. My clients say that meditation brings a feeling of calm – something many haven't felt for years, except on holiday. With meditation you can have that feeling every day!

Give it a go and see how you feel afterwards.

Part 2: Win

The second part of the Stress Shield is simple but powerful.

Many of my clients have negative thoughts and feelings about their fitness. They think it's too hard. That if they haven't lost weight, all the effort is for nothing. Sound familiar?

These negative thoughts can erode your motivation until eventually you give up. You need to conquer them for long-term success. But that can be hard, especially if you have struggled with your weight for years. That negative voice can be so powerful it can seem impossible to get past. This hasn't happened by accident. It arises because that negativity has become the dominant voice in your head, forcing your positive encouraging voice to become shy and weak. You can change this with a simple daily technique grounded in science. Let's look first at how that negative voice has become so powerful.

Imagine your mind is a bank with two cashiers where, instead of withdrawing money, you withdraw thoughts. Whenever anything goes wrong, you go straight to the negative thoughts cashier in your mind bank to withdraw your whole account of negative thoughts. You never visit the positive thoughts desk. Over time, the negative cashier can see you coming and already has a stack of negative thoughts ready for you. Meanwhile, the positive thoughts cashier gets very little practice at dishing out positive thoughts. Because of that, they aren't good at it and have become lazy.

It's not that we want to be overly positive all the time. That too can lead to emotional eating – when things are going well, the 'I deserve a treat' mentality creeps in. We want to have a balanced approach that will help you make a non-emotional decision on what to do next. One based on logic rather than pure emotion.

In my programmes, we use two tools as part of the Stress Shield process to reach that state. We start with the daily win. It's simple. All you need to do is write down one 'win' – one thing that went well from the past 24 hours.

This works because what you focus on grows. If you only focus on things that don't work, these negative thoughts will build up and you will feel despondent and demotivated and before long you'll give up. To have a more balanced view of what is really going on, and to achieve a calm and productive mindset, you need to start deliberately focusing on the positives.

Let's say your weight has gone up one pound despite sticking to your diet and exercise regime. What possible 'wins' could you take from this situation instead? Maybe you stuck to the programme regardless of what the number said on the scales, or you finished a project at work and only gained one pound instead of the usual half a stone. The point is to proactively look for things that are working because that makes us feel good. Then you are more likely to continue and see that little blip on the scales drop down again, rather than throw in the towel and really cause some damage.

Using the daily win strategy will help you feel good and get yourself into a productive mindset every single day. But there's one more tool inside the Stress Shield that is even more powerful. We call this the Thought Transformer.

Part 3: Thought Transformer

What do you do when you are stressed out and feeling overwhelmed – comfort eat, order a takeaway, open a bottle of wine, gorge on cheese or chocolate? These are not ideal if you want to lose weight. But this stress hasn't come from nowhere. It is usually triggered by external events such as an issue at work or at home. It could be your own behaviour such as skipping a workout or seeing that your weight has gone up a pound or two on the scales.

We can't stop these events from happening. They are an inevitable part of life. But they can lead to undesirable consequences such as giving up until next Monday, eating and drinking too much or skipping workouts.

While we can't always control what's happening around us, we can control our reaction to it. By understanding this, you can completely change the trajectory of your fitness journey. In between an event occurring and the actions you take, there is a series of thoughts and emotions. These happen so quickly and the patterns have been repeated so many times that they take place almost unconsciously. When an event occurs, we place our own unique filter or perspective on it. Byron Katie, the bestselling author of *Loving What Is*, calls this perspective a 'story'.[12]

Just as you can now add thousands of different filters to a photo you take on your phone, and each filter will make that photo look subtly but noticeably different, we put our own filters on every situation or event we come across. My client Shirley was a good example of this.

CASE STUDY: SHIRLEY

My client Shirley recently became a grandmother but her daughter was involved with the wrong crowd and wasn't looking after her baby properly. Understandably, this was a worrying situation for Shirley. Shirley's original perspective (or story), whenever she received bad news about her granddaughter, was: 'I need a drink.' As a consequence, she opened a bottle of wine most evenings and, despite working out four or five times a week, the wine caused her to steadily gain weight. But Shirley felt entitled to that bottle of wine. She felt stressed, worried, anxious, upset and afraid. Those feelings and emotions lead to an action which, when repeated day after day, week after week, made it impossible for her to get the results she wanted in her life.

Whenever we take an action that sets us back, it doesn't come from nowhere. There is a predictable set of steps we take, based on the perspective or story we create about an event in our life that ultimately leads to the results we get.

The sequence goes like this:

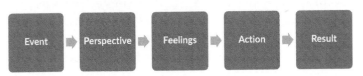

Here's an example of this:

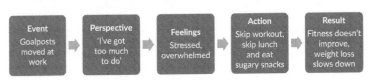

Can you see how the perspective or story we tell about a situation can trigger a sequence of events that can derail us? The more we repeat those stories to ourselves, the more we believe them and the more ingrained the bad habits become.

There is a way to break the cycle, and it starts with challenging those stories you have been telling yourself. I invited Shirley to consider whether her 'I need a drink' story was true. Did she need a drink, or did she just want a drink?

It is a subtly different perspective, but Shirley agreed that while she certainly wanted a drink to quell her anxiety and worry, she didn't need it. In fact, she conceded the drink gave her hot flushes at night, disrupting her sleep, and she never woke up feeling refreshed. That meant her energy levels were low and she fell behind at work, which added to the stress and overwhelm.

What happened next was remarkable. Shirley stopped drinking. She flipped her perspective from 'I need a drink' to 'I want a drink' to 'I don't want a drink', and eventually to 'I need to find a better way to manage the stress in my life'. She started doing yoga every evening instead, and because she was no longer drinking, the weight started to fall off. While the challenges were still there with her daughter and granddaughter, she took them all in her stride.

This process of flipping your original perspective to an opposite perspective, eg 'I need a drink' to 'I don't need a drink', is something we do in our programmes using the Thought Transformer. Initially we apply this to fitness problems, but often clients use it for family and work challenges too. That is the beauty of the Thought Transformer – it can change every aspect of your life and it only takes 5 minutes a day to complete.

So that you can experience this for yourself, I've developed a bonus online training and a Thought Transformer template for you. You can access these at www.trinitytransformation.co.uk/thoughttransformer. You will find out how to use the Thought Transformer to manage the stress in your life better, get your head in the right place every day and stay motivated to achieve all your fitness and life goals.

Reflection

You can experience a taste of the power of the Stress Shield process right now by completing just one of the elements – the win. By focusing on what is working in our lives, rather than what isn't working, we will immediately feel more positive and motivated.

However, rather than writing down just one win, like we do each day in the Stress Shield, we're going to supercharge it by writing down multiple wins. Look back at the past year and write down every win you can think of, no matter how big or small. This is an exercise I do at the end of every year, and it always blows my mind how much more I've done and achieved than I give myself credit for. I bet you're the same.

One thing that can help is to get out your phone and scroll back through your calendar or photos to remind you of what you've done. Don't hold back – write down everything that comes into your mind and create the longest possible list.

Just imagine if you took the time and energy you used to achieve those things and applied it to becoming fit over forty. With the right approach, support and guidance, just think what you could achieve.

Summary

The key takeaway from this chapter is that we all put our own perspective or story on a situation. It is not the situation or event that leads us to eat, drink or give up on our fitness goals, it is the story we tell *about* the situation that leads to those negative outcomes.

Change the stories you tell and you will change your life. Combine that with the daily win and meditation and you will shield yourself from stress every day, making you an unstoppable force on your quest to become fit over forty.

The Stress Shield is the last key puzzle piece that, combined with LIST, the Diet Makeover and age and hormone-specific nutrition targets, means clients on my programmes are able to lose 1–2 stone in 12 weeks, where previously they struggled to lose more than a couple of pounds.

10
Lifestyle

We've now covered three key areas of the Fit Over 40 programme – exercise, nutrition and mindset. If you get these right and do them consistently, the weight will fall off, you'll tone up all over and be back into your favourite clothes in no time – you might even need an entire new wardrobe a size smaller.

However, if there is a fundamental issue with your lifestyle, sticking to the process can be impossible. When that happens, you need to identify and revamp those areas to give you the right platform to succeed.

In this chapter, we will look at each lifestyle factor in turn and why it is so difficult to succeed if it's not right. I'll then give you simple tactics to rectify it.

Sleep

Sleep is essential, not only to be healthy, but also to put your body into a state where it's easy to lose weight quickly. Poor sleep is now ranked as the second biggest cause of obesity, after poor nutrition and *before* exercise. Lack of sleep severely disrupts the key hunger hormones leptin and ghrelin. These hormones work in tandem to control your appetite. Ghrelin drives hunger and cravings. When someone doesn't get enough sleep, ghrelin increases, making their cravings stronger. Leptin controls satiety – the feeling of fullness. If you haven't slept enough, levels of leptin fall, meaning that when you do eat you don't feel full and often want more.

Research has found that the foods people tend to crave when sleep deprived are sweet and salty foods which contain lots of calories, rather than healthy filling foods like proteins and vegetables. This means that when sleep deprived you have to constantly battle against your cravings, which are most likely for fattening high-calorie foods. Even then, you won't feel full and will continue to eat and drink far more than you need. Matthew Walker, bestselling author of *Why We Sleep*, says that 'lack of sleep is the perfect recipe for obesity'.[13]

The amount of sleep you get also changes *how* your body loses weight. Walker describes how researchers studied the difference in weight loss between two groups. The first group, who slept 5 hours a night, lost 70% of their weight from muscle, not from body fat.

The second group, who slept 8 hours a night, lost more than 50% from body fat, meaning they lost weight from those flabby problem areas. Even if they lost exactly the same amount of weight on the scales, which is unlikely, the group who slept properly would end up leaner and more toned than the group who were sleep deprived.

How much sleep is enough? Research tells us that humans need 8 hours' sleep a night to function properly. Matthew Walker says that even 7 hours is not enough: 'Humans need more than seven hours of sleep each night to maintain cognitive performance. After ten days of just seven hours of sleep, the brain is as dysfunctional as it would be after going without sleep for twenty-four hours.'

Walker explains that the amount of sleep someone needs does not decrease with age. Although many people struggle to sleep as they get older, their body still requires 8 hours' sleep to work properly, and not getting it is one of the primary reasons that a lot of people's mental and physical health deteriorates so quickly as they get older.

However, if you're not sleeping enough, it's likely some other element of your lifestyle is disrupting your sleep and therefore your weight loss. Let's dive into some other key lifestyle factors which can ruin your sleep and your weight loss.

Caffeine

One of the main reasons for disrupted sleep is caffeine. Caffeine is the most widely consumed psychoactive drug in the world, largely due to its mood-enhancing and stimulatory effects.[14] Many of my clients are reliant on caffeine before we start working together. This dependency tends to increase over the years as they progress in their careers and their workload becomes more demanding.

Caffeine can make you feel more alert and focused, but it's important to understand how it achieves this and to know the side effects. It helps you feel more awake by blocking a molecule called adenosine. This molecule helps you wind down and get to sleep. Adenosine is produced primarily from physical work and intensive brain use. It binds to receptors in our brain, and the more adenosine accumulates in your brain each day, the more tired you will feel. When we consume caffeine, the caffeine molecules bind to the same receptors in our brain that adenosine attaches to, preventing us from feeling tired.

The downside is that caffeine molecules have a half-life of between 3 and 10 hours depending on your genetics, with an average of around 6 hours. That means it takes 6 hours for your body to break down just half of the caffeine in your system. If you drink a cup of coffee at 4pm, at 10pm you will still have quite a bit of caffeine in your system and won't feel tired.

It becomes a vicious cycle. You have caffeine to help you through the day but your sleep becomes more disrupted, your energy levels fall and you become reliant on caffeine to mask that tiredness.

My recommendation is to consume caffeine in the morning only. It *can* help you feel more alert, and you don't have to stop entirely. But if you need several coffees in the afternoon, you are masking a more serious problem – that you're not sleeping properly. Caffeine can't fix any of the other side effects of sleep deprivation. Your cravings will still be through the roof, you won't feel full even after eating, and you'll feel weak when exercising (or not want to do it altogether) which will make it difficult to lose or maintain your weight.

Alcohol

Alcohol is one of the main reasons women I speak to struggle to get the scales moving. I'm not going to tell you to stop drinking, but to see good results this must be in moderation because alcohol is high in calories.

It contains seven calories per gram. For context, carbs and protein only contain four calories per gram. Only dietary fat is higher, at nine calories per gram. So the calorie content of alcohol is much higher than carbs and closer to fat. Also, because alcohol is a liquid, it is easy to consume large amounts of it. A bottle of wine contains over 600 calories. That's the equivalent of eating three large jacket potatoes!

Not only is alcohol high in calories, but it also causes an increase in appetite and lowers your inhibitions. When you've had a few drinks, you crave high-calorie comfort foods like crisps, salted nuts, cheese or chocolate and you lose the ability to say no. It's not just the calories in alcohol itself that are the problem, it's also the calories from everything else consumed after drinking that start to stack up fast, and your ability to resist those things goes out the window. But that's only the start.

Alcohol also severely disrupts sleep quality. It can help you drift off, but once asleep you will struggle to achieve a quality night's sleep. Even without a hangover, a poor night's sleep after drinking will disrupt the sleep hormones leptin and ghrelin, leading to worse cravings and, in most cases, consuming a lot more calories throughout the next day.

On top of that, poor sleep caused by even moderate alcohol consumption will mean energy levels will be low the next day, making it more likely you will seek out sugary snacks as a pick-me-up. So, as you can see, alcohol can quickly start to make losing weight difficult.

So how much can you drink and still see good progress? The optimum is one or two drinks once or twice a week. Any more can easily become a slippery slope. Of course, not all drinks are created equal. Some are much higher in calories than others. The lowest calorie choice is a single shot of a spirit with a diet mixer, for example a single slimline gin and tonic. This has around 55–60 calories per drink.

In contrast, a large glass of wine is 190–210 calories depending on the type of wine. This means you can have three single G&Ts and it's still fewer calories than just one large glass of wine. Another relatively low calorie choice is champagne or prosecco, which has around 85–90 calories per glass. This is partly because it is carbonated and partly because a champagne flute is a lot smaller than a wine glass, but it does mean you can have two glasses of champagne or prosecco to one large glass of wine. While cocktails are tempting, they are loaded with alcohol and sugar. Some cocktails are over 500 calories per drink, which is the equivalent of a whole meal in every drink, so they're best avoided when trying to lose weight.

For most people, making these compromises with alcohol is enough. If you are an all-or-nothing person when it comes to alcohol, it will be far easier to cut alcohol out entirely while focusing on losing weight. Then you can reintroduce it once you've lost the weight.

Finally, like caffeine, alcohol makes many of the side effects of menopause worse, especially hot flushes, so it's best to keep it to a minimum if you want to feel better during perimenopause and menopause.

Hobbies, fun and 'me time'

Many of our clients spend years climbing the career ladder and building a family, but this hasn't left much time for themselves. They have few hobbies and very little 'me time' to speak of. This might seem irrelevant when it comes to getting fit over forty, but it is more closely linked than you think.

If your life is all about work, chores and family responsibilities, and without any planned 'me time' or fun, your mind will turn to the easiest possible source of fun and excitement available you. In most cases, that's food and drink.

CASE STUDY: BECKY

This is exactly what my client Becky did before joining our Fit Over 40 programme. She has two young children and works at a senior level in a demanding global role. Her free time was filled with family responsibilities.

However, she was constantly stressed and, by the end of the week, she couldn't wait for a takeaway and a bottle of wine. Her weight was at an all-time high, having gained 10 kg (1 st 8 lbs) since getting married, and now in her forties, nothing she tried seemed to get the scales moving.

Becky used our F3 Formula to get back some 'me time'. She and her husband both decided to take an evening off when the other partner would watch the kids, and vice versa. On Becky's evenings, she'd go on a walk with a friend, do a yoga class or go to a café with a good book. She felt so relaxed afterwards that she no longer needed a huge takeaway or a couple of bottles of wine to cope. She didn't stop drinking entirely, and although she ordered a takeaway from time to time, she made healthier choices and met the nutrition targets I'd given her.

Becky lost 10 kg (1 st 8 lbs) and got back to her pre-pregnancy weight in 6 months, and now continues to maintain that weight effortlessly. A big part of that is ensuring her life is in balance across the F3 Formula – fitness, family and fun. Becky realised that rest, relaxation, fun and 'me time' were needed for exceptional performance at work and at home.

'Me time', fun, rest and relaxation are key parts of the success of the F3 Formula. Some members do online art classes, dressmaking or knitting, yoga, swimming, running (in moderation) or cycling. Some have taken up netball, ice skating, singing or horse riding, often hobbies they did when they were younger.

In all cases, my clients have found it easier to stay consistent and avoid giving in to temptation with food and drink when they have something else to look forward to and get excited about each week.

This is a tricky concept for many mothers, especially with younger children. Guilt stops them taking time for themselves away from the family. This is why it's important to have quality time planned with the family too.

Many women I work with find it hard to put themselves first. They feel they are selfish or a bad parent by taking that time away from the family. But there is a big difference between spending time with someone and spending *quality* time with someone. It's easy to spend countless hours with the family without any of it being quality time. Spending quality time with someone means you *consciously* give them your full attention for a period of time, usually one on one.

If you do this deliberately each week, you will have guilt-free 'me time' because you *know* the needs of your loved ones have been met.

Overworking

Overworking causes many of my clients to struggle with their weight. Modern western culture has created a generation of people who are overworked, overweight, overtired and constantly turning to food and drink to cope. The problem with this is two-fold.

Firstly, it creates a sedentary lifestyle. We know that the key to losing weight is consuming the right number of calories for you, and that must take into account your general level of activity. If you spend all day tied to your desk, your activity level will be low. This means you need a low number of calories just to maintain your weight, let alone lose weight.

You may decide to eat less. However, that can feel impossible to stick to if you are overworked as your hormones will be working against you. Cortisol, the stress hormone, makes it harder to lose weight. If it's constantly elevated, because you are overworked and burned out, you'll be battling against leptin resistance, insulin resistance and thyroid deregulation.

To see good progress, you must manage stress levels and hormones – you need a balance. You can do *anything*, but you can't do *everything*. If you want to lose weight over forty, you must prioritise your health and fitness. It doesn't mean you need to quit your job but it does mean changing the way you operate.

Secondly, your capacity to work effectively is linked to your health and fitness. If you don't get enough sleep, don't exercise and drink too much, how effective are you being with your work?

My clients find their clarity, energy levels and productivity go through the roof as soon as they get a handle on their health and fitness, which means they can stop working until 10pm and get back to a healthy work-life balance because they get more done during the day.

CASE STUDY: LOU

Lou worked over 50 hours a week in a demanding job leading a team of scientists. Her weight had reached an all-time high. She struggled to fit into size 20s. Her back ached and her joints hurt. Her energy levels were at rock bottom. Lou realised that stress was a huge contributing factor to her unhealthy lifestyle. She re-evaluated her life and joined my programme. Since then, Lou has lost over 7 stone (44 kg) and has ditched her size 20s for size 10s. Her BMI has gone from over 40, which is classed as severely obese, to under 22, well within the healthy range. She now says she feels like a different person and her energy for life is back. She's no longer hiding behind unflattering clothes and she feels confident again.

You can see Lou's results and in-depth interview about how she achieved all that at www.trinitytransformation.co.uk/results.

This holistic approach of our Fit Over 40 programme ensures our clients' entire lifestyle is set up to achieve their weight loss goals.

In the next chapter, I'll walk you through the process we go through with our clients to set goals that ensure they are motivated and have a clear path to follow to get fit over forty.

Reflection

A mentor of mine said: 'The quality of your life comes down to the quality of the questions you ask yourself.' I have found this to be true for myself and my most successful clients.

Here are questions I use with my clients to help improve their lifestyle:

1. How many units of alcohol do you drink per week? What would be the ideal outcome for you with alcohol?

2. How many caffeinated drinks do you drink a day (tea, coffee, energy drinks)? What would be the ideal outcome for you with caffeine?

3. How many hours of quality sleep do you get a night? What would be the ideal outcome for you when it comes to sleep?

4. How much quality time do you spend with your significant other? What would be the ideal outcome for you when it comes to your significant other?

5. How many hours do you work per week, on average? What would be the ideal outcome for you when it comes to working hours?

Summary

It's essential to make sure your lifestyle supports the goals you're aiming for with your fitness.

You can do anything, but you can't do everything. You can only have so many top priorities in your life, and you will struggle to succeed with your fitness goals if you're working 60-hour weeks and not prepared to change it.

You must have a balance between work, family life and me time, or they will steamroller your best intentions to eat well and exercise.

It's also critical to make sure caffeine and alcohol are consumed in moderation, otherwise they will ruin your sleep. Getting 7–8 hours' quality sleep a night is essential for keeping cravings at bay and maintaining motivation. Sacrifice your sleep and you'll be making it ten times harder to lose weight.

11
Goal-Getting

Before you put the Fit Over 40 process into action, it's important to have clear goals to motivate you and keep you going. Most people put little thought into setting goals and the process behind it, which sets them up to fail before they've started.

In this chapter, I'll teach you the goal-getting process I've perfected over the past decade, which has been proven to work for myself and thousands of my clients. I call it goal-getting, not goal-setting, because this process is about creating something you'll actually achieve, rather than a fantasy goal you set and then quickly forget.

The problem with most goals is that they are too vague to be measurable. If your goal is to lose a bit of weight, how do you know if you're on or off track? You'll quickly feel demoralised, no matter how much weight you've lost, because it can feel like you're failing if you have nothing to measure your progress against.

However, even if you do have a SMART (specific, measurable, achievable, realistic and time-bound) goal, it still probably won't cut it for weight loss. One of my mentors said: 'Those that succeed and those that fail have the same goals,' and it's true. Many of my clients want to lose weight and by a certain date – they all have a SMART goal, but some succeed while others barely lose anything. Why?

This comes down to what I call 'tripwires'. In between where you are now and your goal, there is a series of barely visible tripwires waiting to catch you out. When most people set a new weight loss goal, they wander blindly forwards and do the same things they've always done, hoping for a different outcome. This almost never works, and they quickly stumble into the first tripwire. It might be someone suggesting a takeaway after a stressful week or an office drinks party. There are hundreds of tripwires like these, and most people give up after hitting the first few.

It is possible to spot these tripwires in advance and put strategies in place to defuse them before they become a problem. In this chapter, I'll tell you about the goal-getting process I use with members of my programmes. For most people, goal-setting is a waste of time. They think about what they'd like to achieve but know deep down they won't achieve it. Then they make the goal small and vague, such as 'I just want to lose a bit of weight', which is neither exciting or motivating, and ultimately pointless.

The goal-getting exercise I'm about to walk you through may take a little longer, but you will create powerful goals that will motivate you, and provide a clear roadmap to make those goals a reality as quickly and easily as possible by dodging the tripwires along the way.

The goal-getting process

Most people rush into setting goals and aim for targets that are far-fetched 'pie in the sky' aims that can be more demotivating than motivating. They often end up setting goals that pull in opposite directions.

My client Fiona had recently started a new job and was working from 9am to 11pm most nights. On top of this, she decided to sell her house and build a new dream home with her husband as well as lose weight and get back to her pre-pregnancy shape. This was a recipe for disaster. She had too many top priorities in her life at once and she had left zero time for exercise and looking after her health and fitness. The problem was that she wanted to achieve three different big life goals that all pulled in different directions. As she focused more on her work, her health and happiness suffered.

It is better to create goals that are aligned together and that push you in the same direction. The goal-getting process will help you develop your dreams into simple, realistic, measurable goals that pull in the same direction. Your goals then feel achievable, and you feel motivated to move towards them.

The first step is not to think about the goals, but instead to think about the starting point – where you are today. If you are not crystal clear on this, you may set goals in areas that won't improve your life or, as in Fiona's case, goals that actually make it more stressful and less enjoyable. Figure out your current situation, to come up with a plan to get to where you want to be.

To do this we use our TRINITY Target. Here you rate a number of key areas of your life out of ten, so that you can quickly and easily see the areas where there are problems and which require the most improvement.

These key areas start with the F3 Formula – fitness, family and fun – and then we break each of these down into sub-categories such as health, confidence, relationships with your partner or children and so on. You can download an example of the TRINITY Target from www.trinitytransformation.co.uk/goalgetting.

Start by working around the circle clockwise and put a cross in each area. The inside of the circle is a rating of zero out of ten, meaning that area of your life couldn't be worse, and a cross on the outside of the circle represents a rating of ten out of ten, meaning that area of your life couldn't be better. Once you've worked your way around the circle, connect the crosses and shade in the middle area, just like the example below.

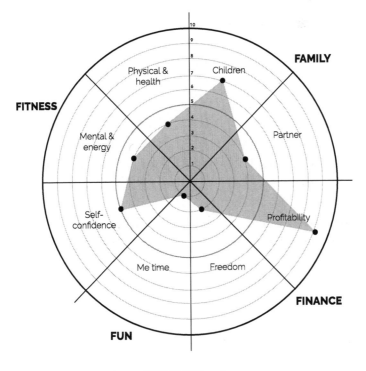

TRINITY Target

Your TRINITY Target will quickly show you the areas of your life that are not working well, along with those that are working effectively. This can be a powerful reality check, as often we continue to push more and more in areas that are already working well while we avoid working on problem areas that will only get worse.

Once you've filled out the TRINITY Target, highlight your bottom three areas – these are the areas with the lowest scores. Don't judge yourself based on these ratings. Use this as inspiration to change it. This process will bring clarity to what is and isn't working in your life and give you direction with what to prioritise moving forwards.

Next, write down the facts in these three lowest rated areas. For example, if you rated your physical fitness as four out of ten, what are the facts about physical health and fitness in your life? These facts are all things you can measure. They are not subjective, they are objective. For example, instead of writing 'I work out occasionally', quantify it: 'I work out once a week'.

You will then end up with a list of facts in each area, like this:

- Age: 47

- Weight: 14 stone 3 lbs (90 kg)

- Menopausal, no HRT

- Dress size: 16

- One workout a week at most

- 3,500 steps a day average

- Drink alcohol 3 days a week

These facts are all important as they will give you a clear idea of your starting point and, when you review your goals, you can measure whether you have improved or not.

Don't skip this step, even if it feels uncomfortable, as it will be difficult to gauge how successful you've been with your goals. If it is uncomfortable, it's not a bad thing. You can use that feeling as motivation to do something about it – being fed up is a good motivator to change something.

As Tony Robbins says, 'Change happens only when the pain of staying the same is greater than the pain of change.'[15] Don't hide from your current reality if it's a bit painful, as feeling that pain wholeheartedly is what will motivate you to actually do something about it. Now you have a clear starting point, it's time for the fun bit – setting your goals.

This can be done by answering one powerful question: 'If we were having this conversation in a year's time, what would you like your life to look like?' Don't hold back here. It's easy to set a goal, then change it for something that seems easier, and to keep doing this until the goal is boring. I see this with clients all the time.

My client Sophie was divorced and wanted to find a life partner. Her initial goals were safe – tiny improvements on her existing life. I asked Sophie to go away and dream big about her goals. She came back with a completely different list, goals that truly excited her and motivated her to make some real changes.

You don't have to set wild goals in every area of your life, but don't make them boring because you're not sure how to get there. We'll get to how to change that shortly.

Your goals have to be in alignment. It wouldn't make sense to set the following goals for the year:

- Lose 4 stone

- Quit my job and start a new business

- Raise our newborn twins

- Move house

- Go on four all-inclusive holidays

These goals are pulling in different directions. Starting a business and raising young children takes time and energy. Moving house is one of the most stressful things anyone can do, and all-inclusive holidays are all about eating and drinking your money's worth. These things make prioritising your health and fitness enough to lose 4 stone almost impossible.

These goals, on the other hand, all fit nicely together:

- Lose 4 stone

- Turn our garage into a home gym I love to be in

- Work maximum 40 hours a week, never at weekends

- Quit being a trustee

- Reconnect with my husband

I'd recommend writing three to five top goals for the next 12 months. If you come up with more, review your list and circle the five that are most important to you.

Then you need to figure out how to achieve those goals. It's important to break down those long-term goals, otherwise it can seem like an impossible mountain to climb, and when that happens, you'll get overwhelmed and do nothing. Break down long-term goals into simple daily and weekly habits to make your targets a reality.

The following is an example of a weight loss goal:

Daily habits:

- Track everything I eat in advance of eating it

- Do at least 5,000 steps

Weekly habits:

- Check in with my coach to keep accountable and discuss anything I'm struggling with

- Plan my food for the week every Sunday

- Plan when I'll do my three workouts after planning my food

- Prepare my breakfasts for the week on Sunday night

- Drink alcohol one night a week only

You can then add the daily and weekly habits for your other goals.

These may seem insignificant, but these simple actions will help you achieve long-term weight loss success and get you fit over forty. Losing weight is about consistently doing the little things and the big goal will take care of itself. This is the power of daily habits. Ordinary actions done consistently achieve extraordinary results.

However, we have to consider those tripwires we mentioned earlier. They will continue to trip you up unless you plan ahead and devise strategies to deal with them in advance.

The last question I ask when setting goals with my clients is this: 'What do you need to stop doing to make these goals a reality?' Look back over your top five goals and think about everything you do (or don't do) that stops you achieving them.

It could look something like this:

I need to stop:

- Trying to do it all on my own
- Hiding away when I'm struggling
- Pretending the snacks I buy are for the kids, when I know I eat a lot of them
- Denying the impact my weight has on my happiness
- Focusing on doing gym classes and cardio that no longer work over forty
- Winging it with my diet
- Starving myself in the day and bingeing in the evenings
- Letting little niggling injuries stop me doing any form of exercise
- Giving up after 2 weeks

Consider how you can solve these problems. For example, if you need to stop giving up after 2 weeks, perhaps work closely with a coach who checks in with you every week and gives you the accountability to see it through to the end.

This step is critical to ensure you don't fall into the same old traps. Write down all the things that usually stop you and a solution to every step, and then you're almost set to succeed with your top five goals.

Then 'supercharge' those goals. You can do this in two ways.

Leverage

Leverage means 'the exertion of force by means of a lever'.[16] A lever helps someone lift or move something bigger than they could on their own. Leverage with your goals allows you to achieve things you wouldn't normally be able to do on your own. Many people will try to do a fitness programme as cheaply as possible, either investing a few pounds in a cheap fitness app or trying to do it on their own for free. This is a false economy, because they spend years struggling to see real results. If you have a more substantial amount to lose financially, you are more likely to stick to it closely. Every time I have invested in coaching or mentoring, it's been expensive but, not only has it has been better than anything free or cheap, I've also had the leverage to stick to it closely.

Another form of leverage is peer pressure, which is usually not seen as a positive, but can be used to our advantage. Publicly declaring our goals can create a lot of leverage, as we don't want to fail in front of others. Our clients find it useful to share their goals within our Fit Over 40 community, where others on the same path can see it. This creates more accountability, another powerful method to 'supercharge' your goals.

Accountability

Accountability is all about having someone who will be on your case if you are slacking. If things don't go well with achieving your fitness goals, without any accountability you can quietly give up on them and no one will know. This approach will only make the problem worse as your self-belief will dwindle, which is the last thing you want.

The best form of accountability is to find someone you don't know but who you trust can help you achieve the results you want. If it's a friend or family member, you may not take their advice and it can even cause you to do the opposite of what you need to do, just to prove a point. That's why it usually works best to find someone outside your circle of friends and family to keep you accountable.

My team and I hold our clients accountable by monitoring their actions. They check in with us every week, and if they don't, we follow up with them so they see it through to the end no matter what. This high-level accountability is one of the reasons many of our clients see faster results within 12 weeks of starting than they had done for many years.

CASE STUDY: SARAH

You may remember my client Sarah, who we met in Chapters 6 and 7. Before we started working together, I took Sarah through my goal-getting process on the phone. Sarah says setting her goals was critical for her transformation:

'I have taken ownership of my life and that started with writing down goals and really knowing who you are and what your values are. The programme has changed my approach massively. I know what my values are, I know what I want my friendships to be. It is so much more than my weight. While I've lost over 45 pounds (20 kg), it wasn't even really about the weight. I have a routine now; routine is important to me and I've realised that. I need consistency, I need support and accountability. That works for me. It's why the programme worked for me.'

Sarah started by setting clear goals, and combining these with the right accountability and support she was able to achieve more than she ever thought possible.

Reflection

I'd recommend you spend time now going through the goal-getting process, outlined above.

Start by completing your TRINITY Target and highlight your bottom three areas for improvement.

Then answer the following five questions:

1. What are the facts about your life in each of the three areas of the F3 Formula: Fitness, Family and Fun?

2. In twelve months' time, what must have happened for you to be happy with your progress?

3. What daily and weekly habits do you need to have in place to make these goals a reality?

4. What do you need to stop doing in order to make these goals a reality?

5. What leverage (accountability and support) do you need in order to guarantee you achieve these goals?

Take some time to really think about these answers and write them out in a journal or notepad. If you're unsure about any aspect of this process, or you'd like a member of my team to take you through this process,

you can do just that at www.trinitytransformation.
co.uk/goalgetting.

Summary

To feel motivated and focused on your fitness journey, it's important to have clear goals, but not just in the area of fitness – in all areas of your life.

These goals should be specific, measurable and realistic, but they should also be in alignment and not pull you in different directions. They should be complimentary, so achieving one goal also helps in some way towards some of your other goals.

You also need to consider the 'tripwires' you will encounter on the way to achieving those goals and plan how you'll overcome them.

Accountability and leverage are two powerful ways to 'supercharge' your goals and make them easier to achieve.

Don't play your goals down and make them smaller than they need to be. Members of my programme typically lose 1–2 pounds a week, and this adds up to big results over time.

Dream big. The Fit Over 40 programme described in this book is proven to work for thousands of women just like you. Combine that with the support and accountability you need and that dream will become a reality, just like it did for Lou, Sarah, Julie and all the other women whose stories you've heard.

You've got this!

Conclusion

You now understand the process to beat over forty weight gain. It's worked for thousands of women on our programmes and it will work for you, as long as you put it into action.

Knowledge is power, but only if you put it into action. Don't waste the knowledge you've learned in this book. It has the power to transform every aspect of your life, get the scales moving and send your energy through the roof, which will mean you can slip back into your favourite clothes and feel amazing wearing anything you like.

Just think where that energy and confidence could lead. How could it affect your existing relationship, or your ability to find the person you want to spend the rest of your life with? What effect could it have on your career? How would you behave differently with your children, friends and family?

It's time to get the real 'you' back. It won't always be easy, but it will be worth it, and it starts by taking that first step. Don't put it off any longer – it's time to stop wishing and start doing.

Next steps

This book holds everything you need, but it isn't always easy to do alone. If you'd like help making it happen, I'd love to assist you. My team at TRINITY Transformation has spent the past decade working with over 6,500 women to help them get fit over forty and we'd love you to be our next success story.

We offer a free no-obligation discovery call, and on that call a member of our team will take you through our goal-getting process so you'll come away with an action plan and the motivation to get started. You can find out more about my programmes and see more success stories at www.trinitytransformation.co.uk/ programme.

References

1   Y He et al, 'The transcriptional repressor DEC2 regulates sleep length in mammals', *Science*, 325/5942 (2009), 866–870

2   L Newson, *Menopause: All you need to know in one concise manual* (JH Haynes & Co Ltd, 2019)

3   R Holiday, *The Obstacle is the Way: The ancient art of turning adversity to advantage* (Profile Books, 2015)

4   A Ishaya, *200%: An instruction manual for living fully* (Thread of Souls, 2018)

5   C Duhigg, *The Power of Habit: Why we do what we do, and how to change* (Random House Books, 2013)

6   JF Kennedy, 'Remarks in Heber Springs, Arkansas, at the dedication of Greers Ferry Dam'

(1963), www.presidency.ucsb.edu/documents/
remarks-heber-springs-arkansas-the-dedication-
greers-ferry-dam, accessed 22 July 2021

7   L McDonald, *The Women's Book: A guide
to nutrition, fat loss, and muscle gain* (Lyle
McDonald, 2017)

8   A Sharma et al, 'Exercise for mental health', *The
Primary Care Companion to The Journal of Clinical
Psychiatry*, 8/2 (2006), 106

9   P Mort, *Paul Mort Talks Sh*t Podcast: Episode 5 –
James Smith* (2021)

10   M Hallsworth & H Harper, 'Counting
calories: how under-reporting can explain the
apparent fall in calorie intake', www.bi.team/
publications/counting-calories-how-under-
reporting-can-explain-the-apparent-fall-in-
calorie-intake, accessed 22 July 2021

11   D Ford, *Why Good People Do Bad Things: How to
stop being your own worst enemy* (HarperOne, 2009)

12   B Katie, *Loving What Is: Four questions that can
change your life* (Rider, 2002)

13   M Walker, *Why We Sleep: The new science of sleep
and dreams* (Penguin, 2018)

14   K Patel, 'Caffeine', https://examine.com/
supplements/caffeine, accessed 22 July 2021

15   T Robbins, 'Read these Tony Robbins quotes to
prime you for success', www.tonyrobbins.com/
tony-robbins-quotes, accessed 22 July 2021

16   Oxford English Dictionary, 'Leverage', www.
lexico.com/definition/leverage, accessed 22 July
2021

Acknowledgements

Thank you to my co-founder at TRINITY Transformation, Ben Hughes, for making this possible. Without Ben funding the first year of our business, working in a job he didn't enjoy while I worked to get the business off the ground, we would never have been able to get to where we are today, having an impact on thousands of women's lives every year and culminating in writing this book to expand that to thousands more.

To all the amazing members of my programme whose inspiring stories have been shared in this book: Lou Marsh, Sarah Davies, Julie Bates, Patricia Fox, Catherine Muirhead, Caroline Wood, Becky Lepp, Lesley, Sophie, Kerry and Shirley. Thank you for putting your faith in me, my team and the programme, committing wholeheartedly to the Fit Over 40 process and sharing your results with the world to show what is achievable in a healthy way for women over forty. Thank you, too, to all the programme members I haven't had space to mention here – you give my life purpose and I never tire of hearing about your successes.

Thank you to my mentors. To Paul Mort for inspiring me and showing me how to coach people with a no-nonsense attitude, while still being empathetic and caring deeply. To Arjuna Ishaya, who taught me meditation in a non-woo woo way. To Nick James, Tony and Nicki Vee, Adam Ashburn and the team at Expert Empires, who pushed me to get this book done and out into the world, and helped me to focus on my strengths while giving me words of reassurance when I had a wobble.

Finally, to all those who helped put this book together at Rethink Press, especially Siobhan, who helped halve the length of the book and cut down my waffle without losing anything important – a process I think I'd still be struggling to do a decade from now!

The Author

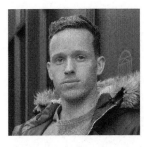 Rob Birkhead is co-founder of TRINITY Transformation and the UK's #1 Health Coach for professional women over forty. He is an expert in sustainable weight loss for women across the areas of exercise, nutrition and mindset, with over a decade's experience working with over 6,500 clients internationally.

Contact Rob and his team:

✉ info@trinitytransformation.co.uk

🌐 www.trinitytransformation.co.uk

f www.facebook.com/trinitytransformation

© @trinitytransformations